VITAMINS &
MINERALS

First published in Great Britain in 2003 by
Hamlyn, a division of Octopus Publishing Group Ltd

This edition published in 2007 by Bounty Books,
a division of Octopus Publishing Group Ltd
2–4 Heron Quays, London E14 4JP

An Hachette Livre UK Company
Reprinted 2008
Copyright © Octopus Publishing Group Ltd 2003

ISBN: 978-0-753716-32-8

A CIP catalogue record for this book is available from the British Library

Printed and bound in China

VITAMINS & MINERALS

Sara Rose

Bounty Books

Contents

A–Z OF SYMPTOMS AND REMEDIES

Introduction

Food and health are intimately connected, and dietary advice is an essential part of healthcare throughout the world. The links between diet and disease have long been recognized, and food has been used as medicine for thousands of years. However, it was not until the 20th century that scientists began to put together a profile of nutrients, including carbohydrates, fats, proteins, vitamins and minerals, essential to health. We now know that without certain vitamins and minerals, metabolism – the process by which the body turns food into energy it can use – simply cannot happen.

Most people today understand what constitutes a healthy lifestyle: stop smoking, drinking alcohol in moderation, exercising regularly and eating a balanced diet that is low in fat, high in fibre and which includes plenty of fresh fruit and vegetables. But putting that advice into practice can be difficult. Furthermore, the stresses and strains of modern living, over which we sometimes have little control, can seriously affect physical and mental wellbeing.

There is strong medical evidence in support of certain specific dietary supplements, including folic acid taken during pregnancy to prevent neural tube defects, and vitamin B[6] to alleviate symptoms of premenstrual syndrome. However, medical opinion about nutrition as a treatment for specific illnesses is more sceptical, except in the cases of gout, high blood cholesterol and diabetes.

How to use this book

This book offers practical advice on vitamins and minerals to help you understand what they do, why you need them and when to take them. The introduction guides you through the basic facts: how vitamins and minerals work and the effects they have on different parts of the body. It explains how your nutritional needs change throughout life and describes the different types of supplements available. The first section of the book, *Essential nutrients*, details the most essential nutrients and how they work in the body. A vital fact panel for each vitamin, mineral or other nutrient provides an instant check on how they help your health, the recommended amounts and the best food sources. The second section, *A–Z of symptoms and remedies*, describes common ailments, and offers guidance on the best nutrients to take to prevent and alleviate symptoms.

Supplements are not intended to replace a healthy, balanced diet, but to ensure your body gets all the nutrients it needs. However, it is important to seek professional advice before self-diagnosing and choosing supplements, and if you are taking any form of medication you should always consult your doctor before taking supplements.

The RDA

Governments around the world have established guidelines on how much of a particular vitamin or mineral we need in our diets. These levels, known as RDAs (recommended daily allowance) or RDIs (recommended daily intake), are standards based on the amounts needed to prevent known nutritional diseases such as beri-beri and scurvy. They are widely regarded as woefully inadequate because they do not exist for a number of key nutrients, do not take into account individual needs and do not reflect new thinking on optimizing health. Those who have a stressful lifestyle, a particular illness or who are on medication, for example, may need much more than the RDA.

How vitamins and minerals work

Nutrients are extracted from the food you eat as it passes through your digestive system. They are essential for cell growth, maintenance and repair; they provide energy to enable your body to function efficiently and to ward off infection and disease. The main nutrients are carbohydrates, fats, proteins, vitamins and minerals. Fibre and water are also essential. No nutrient works alone: each depends on the others to be most effective.

Macronutrients Carbohydrates, proteins and fats are the macronutrients. Carbohydrates and fats provide energy when broken down. Protein provides the building blocks necessary for cell growth and repair.

Carbohydrates Carbohydrates provide the body's basic source of energy. Simple carbohydrates, such as sugars, give instant energy and have no nutritional value. Complex carbohydrates, found in bread, pasta, rice, potatoes, cereals and pulses, release energy slowly and also contain fibre, vitamins and minerals. Wholegrain products are more nutritious than refined products because they are digested slowly, providing sustained energy.

Proteins A daily supply of protein, found in meat, poultry, fish, eggs, nuts, pulses and beans, is essential for cell growth, maintenance and repair. Everybody needs two to three servings of protein per day, but most people in Western cultures eat more protein than they need, which is then converted into fat.

Fats Fats are essential for good health. They insulate your body, cushion vital organs and can be converted into energy. Fats are used to build new cells and are critical for normal brain development and nerve function. There are three categories of fatty acids: saturated fatty acids (SFAs), monounsaturated fatty acids (MUFAs) and polyunsaturated fatty acids (PUFAs). Most fat-containing foods have a balance of all three. There are two types of essential fatty acids (EFAs) in the PUFA category – omega-3 and omega-6 fats – that cannot be made by the body and have to come from your diet. Your body needs EFAs for energy production, building cells, oxygen transport, blood clotting and making extremely active hormone-like substances called prostaglandins.

Micronutrients Vitamins and minerals are micronutrients. They do not in themselves provide energy, but macronutrients depend on them to release energy from food. Vitamins are organic substances. They activate enzymes, which are proteins that act as catalysts to speed up all the biological reactions that take place in your body. Vitamins have important functions in maintaining strong bones and controlling hormonal activity. Your body can make a certain amount of vitamins D and K, but you have to obtain all other vitamins from your diet.

Minerals are inorganic substances that originate from rocks and ores and find their way into the food chain through the soil. We get our minerals either by eating plants grown on mineral-rich soil or by eating animals that have fed on these plants. Calcium, magnesium and phosphorus are the major constituents of bone; sodium and potassium control your body's water balance; and the remaining minerals are needed for various chemical processes to take place in the body.

The digestive system Food passes through the digestive system, where it is broken down by acids and enzymes so that it can be absorbed into the bloodstream and used for energy and to build and repair tissues. The alimentary or digestive canal is a long muscular tube made up of hollow organs such as the stomach and intestines. It extends from the mouth to the anus, and each region specializes in a different stage of food processing. Digestion begins in the mouth but most takes place in the stomach and small intestine. Waste products of digestion are processed by the liver and kidneys and eliminated from the body in the urine and faeces.

The digestion of food and the elimination of waste products are the foundations of good health. If food is not properly digested, you may not be getting all the nutrients you need, and your system may become overloaded with toxins.

Nutrients for optimum health

Study after study has indicated that not only are certain nutrients essential for life, but maximizing your intake of nutrients enables your body to function as efficiently as possible and improves health.

Boosting immunity and fighting infection The best line of defence against illness is to keep your immune system strong so that it is able to fight infection. Inadequate nutrition impairs your body's ability to keep its defences in top working order. Your immune system needs certain vitamins and minerals to produce specialized blood cells that destroy specific invaders. A lack of vitamins A, C and E, and B-complex vitamins, reduces immunity. Vitamin C is crucial for immune system function: it has anti-viral and anti-bacterial properties, and is a natural antihistamine. Essential fats reduce inflammation and infection.

Eating for energy A whole host of nutrients are required to turn food into energy, including most of the B vitamins, vitamin C, iron, copper and magnesium. They help to make hormones, are responsible for nerve transmission and maximize energy.

Weight control Body weight has an effect on health, and every person has an optimal weight linked to their height, bone structure and amount of muscle. Maintaining a healthy weight depends on your ability to burn fat and break down glucose into energy. The B vitamins, vitamin C, iron and chromium are essential for converting glucose into energy and transporting it to the cells. For people who are overweight, supplements of these micronutrients combined with a low-fat, high-fibre diet may help with weight loss. For those who are underweight, zinc and essential fatty acids are thought to play an important role in helping to maintain healthy eating patterns.

Balancing hormones Hormones are powerful chemical messengers that are produced in various glands in the body and carried in the blood to different parts of the body, where they produce a specific effect. For example, insulin, produced in the pancreas, regulates blood sugar levels; and adrenaline, produced by the adrenal glands, co-ordinates your body's response to stress. Hormone production and function is dependent on many vitamins and minerals, particularly vitamin B^3, B^6, biotin, magnesium and zinc, and hormone imbalances cause a wide range of problems from infertility to weight gain. A well-balanced diet, which includes essential fatty acids, will help to keep your hormones in balance.

Healthy heart Heart disease is caused by blood clots, hardening of the arteries to the heart, narrowing of the arteries caused by the build- up of fatty deposits and raised blood pressure. Certain vitamins and minerals have proven benefits for maintaining a healthy heart and blood vessels. Vitamin C helps to keep arteries supple because it is used in the production of collagen, the substance that binds cells together. Increasing your intake of magnesium, potassium and calcium and avoiding adding extra sodium (salt) to your food can reduce blood pressure by helping to relax the blood vessels. Vitamin E and omega-3 fish oils thin the blood, reducing the likelihood of clot formation, and fish oils also help reduce cholesterol (blood fat) levels.

Healthy digestive system A balanced lifestyle and diet are crucial to maintaining a healthy digestive system. Excessive stress, for example, is thought to contribute to poor digestion. If food is not broken down or absorbed properly, it is thought to irritate the lining of the intestines, causing them to become 'leaky'. Food molecules and toxins then pass into the bloodstream, causing problems in other parts of the body, depleting the immune system and leaving you vulnerable to illness. Poorly digested food in the intestines is also thought to upset the intestinal balance, leading to an overgrowth of unfriendly bacteria.

Improving digestion is the key to good health because of the knock-on effects this has on the rest of your body. Vitamin B^6

and zinc are needed to produce digestive enzymes, and calcium and magnesium help to reduce excess stomach acid (which causes indigestion). Acidophilus improves the activity of beneficial bacteria in the intestines.

Strong bones and powerful muscles You need to eat sufficient quantities of calcium, magnesium and phosphorus to keep your bones strong and healthy. Vitamin D controls calcium uptake and is helped by boron. Vitamin C makes collagen, which strengthens connective tissue. If you want to improve your athletic performance, you should increase your intake of vitamins A, C and E. These help your body to detoxify the by-products of metabolism, and increase oxygen uptake into the cells. Co-enzyme Q10 is also important for the transport of oxygen in the body.

Mental health Mental health is a complex area but there are several nutritional factors that are known to influence mood and mental function. For example, your brain needs glucose – the end product of carbohydrate metabolism – to function properly. However, the body's the ability to use glucose depends on several vitamins and minerals, especially vitamins B^3 and B^6, chromium, manganese and zinc. Blood sugar levels, which affect mood, can be unbalanced by consuming too much of the wrong thing, such as caffeine, cigarettes and alcohol.

Looking good Good nutrition is vital to keep your skin looking good. The skin's elasticity depends on collagen, which makes it flexible. Vitamin C is needed to make collagen, and it also neutralizes free radicals that damage the skin and cause wrinkles. Vitamin A is important to keep skin smooth and supple, while vitamin E protects skin cells from damage and encourages skin to heal. Zinc is needed to regenerate skin cells and essential fatty acids keep the skin from drying out.

Retarding the ageing process Research indicates that the ageing process is the result of the body's declining ability to repair the damage caused by free radicals. Increasing your intake of antioxidants, which neutralize free radicals, will help you to look and feel better as you get older.

Free radicals and antioxidants

Much of the cell damage that occurs in disease is caused by destructive chemical groups known as free radicals. These are the products of oxidation, a natural by-product of metabolism, that exist for only a very short period of time. Because there is so much pollution in the air today, there are more free radicals than ever. In small quantities, free radicals can support your immune system by fighting antigens (foreign substances). But in large quantities, they can damage cellular DNA, accelerating the ageing process and contributing to a range of illnesses, and have an effect on cholesterol such that it furs up the arteries.

Free radicals can be neutralized by antioxidants, which seek them out and deactivate them. The main antioxidants are vitamins A, C and E, plus the minerals selenium and zinc, and manganese and copper. Research indicates that increasing your intake of antioxidants can significantly lower the risk of developing heart disease and other serious illnesses.

Top tips for good skin
- Avoid strong sunlight and use sun cream
- Drink at least a litre of water daily
- Limit intake of alcohol, caffeine, nicotine, additives, salt and sugar
- Eat plenty of fresh fruit and vegetables

What nutrients do you need?

There are many factors to take into account when assessing your nutritional status. The nutrients you need vary not only according to your age, sex and general state of health, but also according to your lifestyle. In an ideal world, most people would get all the nutrients they need from their diet alone, but today's pace of life means that taking supplements is sometimes necessary.

Lifestyle and health robbers Stress is a physical or mental demand that causes the body to become flooded with stress hormones, which produce physical changes in the body, such as a pounding heart, sweating and tense muscles. A certain degree of stress is not necessarily a bad thing: it provides the spur to achieve, for example. But long-term stress can cause you to experience symptoms such as headaches and feelings of anxiety even when the source of stress is not there.

Paradoxically, when we are under stress we increase our dependency on stimulants to give us a quick burst of energy, and although these may seem to be effective in the short term, in the long term they have serious implications for health. Stimulants, such as tea, coffee and sugar, are substances that increase physiological activity. Their effect on the body is rather like that of rocket fuel – they give a quick burst of energy followed by a rapid burnout. They boost your energy levels by stimulating the adrenal glands (which sit on top of the kidneys) to release hormones that give your body's cells an express delivery of glucose. You soon become caught in a vicious circle whereby you need more of the stimulant to get the same effect, until you become dependent on it. Stimulants also contain toxins, and your body has only a finite capacity to deal with these. The more stimulants you take, the more your body remains in a state of red alert and you become prey to anxiety, fatigue and mood swings.

Research has indicated that the body uses up more vitamins when under stress, either from illness or daily life. Smoking and drinking alcohol make it harder for the body to absorb vitamins, so if you smoke or drink heavily, you should pay special attention to your diet.

Children A healthy, organic diet should cover the majority of a child's nutritional needs. However, because many children don't eat much red meat, you need to watch out for iron-deficiency anaemia. It is also important to ensure that a child's diet contains sufficient levels of calcium, which is vital for normal bone growth. Fatty acids are crucial for intellectual development, along with vitamins B and C. If you think your child may need to take supplements it is best to seek medical advice to ensure that the products are safe and suitable for children.

Adolescents The physical changes of puberty mean that your child will need extra vitamins A, D and B^6, biotin, zinc, calcium, magnesium and essential fatty acids. These nutrients encourage optimum growth and development and zinc is also essential for sexual maturity.

Your child's weight may increase significantly during adolescence, and you need to watch out for bad eating habits that can lead to excess weight gain and poor health. Make sure your teenager sticks to a healthy diet and eats regularly.

Adults There is considerable evidence to show that eating a healthy diet can improve your general health. Men, in particular, are much more likely to smoke, drink to excess and neglect their health. Heart disease, your response to stress and fertility seem to be very much affected by diet. Key nutrients include antioxidants to deal with the harmful effects of stress and boost immunity, and selenium and zinc for fertility.

Premenstrual syndrome Hormonal imbalances related to the menstrual cycle mean that many women regularly suffer from symptoms such as depression, irritability, water retention, headaches and low energy levels in the time leading up to their monthly periods. Foods containing vitamin B^6, magnesium, zinc and evening primrose oil may all help to alleviate symptoms and maintain hormonal balance.

Pregnancy and breastfeeding Research has shown that pregnant woman need about twice as much protein, iron, calcium and folic acid as women who are not pregnant, and essential fatty acids are crucial for the development of the foetus's brain during pregnancy. You may be advised to take a good multivitamin and multimineral supplement, as it may be difficult to obtain all the nutrients you need through diet alone. Supplements should be specifically designed for pregnancy; for example, you should not take vitamin A supplements while pregnant because an excess of vitamin A can cause birth defects. Breastfeeding also depletes your store of nutrients and you may need extra vitamins and minerals during this period.

It is a good idea for women who plan to have more than one child to ensure they have a well-balanced diet between pregnancies; this is particularly important for women who are vegetarian.

Menopause The menopause puts extra stress on a woman's body because of the falling levels of oestrogen, which can contribute to symptoms such as hot flushes, night sweats, mood swings and loss of bone mass. B vitamins may improve mood; you need extra calcium, magnesium and phosphorus to maintain bone density; and minerals such as zinc and selenium may help to alleviate hot flushes and balance hormone levels.

Old age As you get older, your body becomes less efficient at absorbing nutrients and your immune system becomes less effective. Zinc (for good digestion), vitamins A, C and E (to counteract damage by free radicals), and supplements such as ginkgo biloba may help to maintain physical and mental functioning.

Do you need to improve your diet?
1   Do you smoke?
2   Do you add salt to your food and eat sweets more than twice a week?
3   Do you eat fried foods?
4   Is your fat intake above 30% of your daily calorie intake?

5   Do you eat processed and 'fast' food?
6   Do you eat red meat more than twice a week?
7   Do you drink more than one cup of coffee or three cups of tea a day?
8   Do you drink more than one unit of alcohol a day?
9   Do you rarely eat fresh fruit and vegetables?
10 Do you often skip meals?

If the answer is yes to most or all of the questions above, then your health is likely to suffer. You need to make permanent changes to your lifestyle and diet.

If you answered yes to half of the questions, you can improve your health by getting rid of bad dietary habits.

If you answered no to most or all of the questions, you are on the right track to a long and healthy life.

Healthy eating

Eating a well-balanced diet that includes plenty of fresh fruit and vegetables can make a big difference to your health. It can make you feel much more alert and increase your vitality and vigour. The amount of food you need to eat in a day depends on your age, sex and level of activity.

Foods for optimum nutrition
- Complex carbohydrates should form half your daily diet
- At least five portions of fruit and vegetables a day, preferably organic
- Low-fat dairy foods
- Oily fish at least twice a week
- Olive oil or other monounsaturated fats for cooking and salads
- Plenty of fibre-rich foods
- Fresh foods whenever possible
- Steam vegetables rather than frying or boiling
- Drink enough fluid to keep urine pale – at least 2 litres of water a day to flush out toxins

Foods to limit or avoid
Drink alcohol in moderation, and try to have at least two alcohol-free days a week. Reduce your caffeine intake by limiting tea, coffee, colas and chocolate. Cut back on processed foods, which are loaded with preservatives, colourings and flavourings, and restrict your consumption of red meat and cheese, both of which are high in saturated fat. Reduce your salt intake – use it in cooking only, don't add it at the table. Limit your intake of sugar so that your blood sugar levels remain stable; this will help to avoid mood swings.

Mood foods and cravings: what they mean
Craving a particular food is sometimes the sign of an allergy, but more often than not it is nature's way of letting you know that you are deficient in certain nutrients. A craving for nuts, peanut butter or yeast extract spread may indicate a vitamin B-complex deficiency. If you find yourself reaching for chocolate when you are unhappy or craving starchy or sugary foods, the chances are that your body needs the mood-enhancing chemicals they contain.

Overfed, but undernourished

In an ideal world we would obtain all our nutrients from a balanced diet, but the truth is that although we are consuming more food than ever before, we are getting fewer and fewer of the essential nutrients. This has a lot to do with the way food is grown and produced – food may be nutritionally deficient even before it reaches the shops. Taking an A–Z-style vitamin and mineral supplement is not a replacement for food, but it will help to fill any gaps that may be present in your diet.

Additives and organic foods

Food additives perform many functions, from giving flavour and colour, to preventing food from spoiling. However, some may produce side effects, such as allergic reactions. Food may also contain potentially harmful substances such as growth hormones, antibiotics and pesticides, which can contribute to toxic overload in the body. If you choose organic food, which is grown without chemicals, you will reduce the threat to your health.

Getting the most vitamins and minerals from your food

- Don't cut or wash fruit and vegetables until you are ready to eat them
- Eat the skins of vegetables
- Eat food raw whenever possible
- Eat foods as fresh as possible, and keep them cool and in the dark if you are not going to eat them immediately
- If cooking, use as little water as possible and keep the water for stock
- Do not overcook food
- Cooking in copper pans can destroy folic acid and vitamins C and E

Taking supplements

Most supplements come in a variety of forms, to suit people's different needs, and you should opt for the version you find easiest to take. They are also prepared with varying amounts of the active ingredients, so you should read the label carefully and make sure you understand what you are taking – the ingredient present in the greatest quantity will be listed first. Too much of any one vitamin or mineral may cause health problems, and it is essential to add up your total intake of nutrients if you are combining supplements.

Tablets are the most practical form of supplement because they are easy to store and keep for a long time. **Capsules** are the usual form for fat-soluble vitamins such as vitamin E. They can also be broken apart and applied to the skin. Fat-soluble vitamins (A, D, E and K) are available in dry or water-soluble forms. **Powders** are more potent than tablets or capsules and have no binders, fillers or additives, making them useful for people with allergies. **Liquids** can be mixed into drinks or food. Both powders and liquids are ideal for children and those unable to swallow capsules or tablets.

What else is in supplements?

Supplements may contain other substances along with the active ingredient. The main ones are: **fillers**, which increase the volume of material; **binders**, which bind the components together (without which the tablet would fall apart); **disintegrants**, which help the supplement to dissolve; and **lubricants**, to stop the tablet from sticking to the machine that presses it out. Supplements may also contain preservatives, colourings, flavourings and sweeteners. If you are a vegan or vegetarian, check the product is not derived from animal sources. Gluten-, yeast- and sugar-free supplements are available.

Chelation

'Chelated' is a term that appears on mineral supplements, and it means that the mineral has been combined with another substance to make absorption more efficient. Chelated minerals pass through the stomach more easily, and cannot bind with other substances in the digestive tract that may interfere with absorption. Minerals are thought to be best absorbed when chelated with amino acids.

Time-release supplements

In time-release supplements, also known as sustained and continuous release, the active ingredients are trickled gradually from the tablet rather than released all at once. Time-release formulas are particularly useful for water-soluble vitamins, which are not stored in the body.

When and how to take supplements

The key to deriving benefit from supplements is to take them regularly. and once a day is easiest for most people. The general rule is to take supplements with food, because this is the way they are absorbed most easily, although some vitamins and minerals work best on an empty stomach. The label on a supplement should tell you the best time to take it. Water-soluble vitamins can leave your body as quickly as 2 hours after you have taken them; fat-soluble vitamins stay in the body for about 24 hours.

Overdosing

There is little point in taking more vitamins than your body needs. In the case of water-soluble vitamins, they are simply flushed out. Fat-soluble vitamins will be stored, and over a period of time this can be extremely damaging to health.

Drug-nutrient interactions

Many drugs, from aspirin to contraceptives, interfere with the action of nutrients, and may increase your need for certain nutrients. If you have a medical condition and are taking drugs to control it, it is essential to seek medical advice before taking supplements, because the combination could be dangerous.

Essential nutrients

This section describes all you need to know about vitamins, minerals and other essential nutrients, with brief descriptions of their main functions, and information on the illnesses they can help prevent and the best dietary sources. Recommended daily amounts are given where these have been established, as well as guidelines for the safe maximum dosage.

An introduction to essential nutrients

Our diet needs to include vitamins and minerals in order for our bodies to work properly and to prevent illness. Vitamins and minerals work in conjunction with each other, and taking large doses of any one supplement can upset your body's balance. A good multivitamin and multimineral supplement will ensure you get the correct amount of each nutrient in the right proportions.

Vitamins

These are divided into two groups, according to whether they are soluble in fat or in water. Fat-soluble vitamins are vitamins A, D, E and K, and they can be stored in your body for months or even years. Water-soluble vitamins are the vitamin B complex and vitamin C. Because they dissolve in water they are easily lost from the body in urine, so you need a regular intake. B-complex vitamins also work synergistically, which means they are more potent when taken together than when taken separately. A deficiency of any vitamin will result in specific vitamin deficiency diseases, such as scurvy or pellagra.

Minerals

These are divided into two main groups: major or macro-minerals, such as calcium, magnesium, potassium, sodium and phosphorus, so-called because we need relatively large amounts; and trace minerals, such as copper, chromium and zinc, which are needed in minute quantities. Like vitamins, a deficiency of any mineral may cause illness, but they may also be harmful if taken in large amounts.

Other essential nutrients

There are a number of other food supplements that are now considered to be crucial to good health. This section covers essential fatty acids, amino acids and co-enzyme Q10. Amino acids form the building blocks of all proteins and are essential for life. While many fats are known to be unhealthy, there are others that are essential for body processes to take place and that work to prevent the effects of 'bad' fats in your body, helping to reduce the risk of heart

Vitamin K

Vitamin K, which is essential for blood clotting, does not have its own entry because it should only be supplemented under medical supervision. Vitamin K is manufactured in the gut and is widely available in food, and deficiency is very uncommon (all newborn babies are given a dose of vitamin K to improve blood clotting). Large doses of vitamin K can cause liver damage, jaundice and the breakdown of red blood cells.

disease and the build-up of cholesterol. Co-enzyme Q10 is a substance that helps enzymes, proteins that speed up chemical processes.

Other supplements

There are a number of other food supplements of non-essential nutrients, many of which have properties that appear to be greatly beneficial to health. Some of the most popular ones are described briefly on pages 86–87.

Vitamin A

A fat-soluble vitamin stored in the liver, vitamin A comes in two forms: retinol, found in animal products; and beta-carotene, which your body converts into vitamin A. It has a number of important functions and is essential for healthy skin, eyesight, growth and reproduction.

How it works

Beta-carotene is a powerful antioxidant that destroys free radicals – molecules that damage healthy cells, speed up the ageing process and can cause a number of serious diseases to develop. Vitamin A promotes the growth of strong teeth and bones, and keeps skin healthy. In the eye, vitamin A is essential for the formation of visual purple, a pigment that lets us see in dim light.

Vitamin A is a well-known immune system booster and helps the body to fight infection. It also plays an important role in wound healing.

Deficiency symptoms

- Poor night vision
- Dandruff
- Dry, flaky skin
- Frequent colds or infection
- Mouth ulcers

Remedies

Acne, wrinkles and psoriasis Many face creams contain vitamin A, and drugs derived from vitamin A are used to treat severe acne. As an antioxidant, vitamin A neutralizes free radicals, substances that destroy collagen (essential for the skin's elasticity), and are known to play a role in inflammatory disorders such as psoriasis.

Viral infections Because of its role in strengthening the immune system and improving resistance, vitamin A helps to protect against sore throats, colds and other viral infections, and shortens the duration of such illnesses.

Vitamin A is often referred to as the 'vision vitamin' because of its benefits for sight.

vital facts
Vitamin A

Recommended daily allowance for adults:

800mcg

Main functions:

- Antioxidant
- Boosts immunity
- Essential for vision
- Healthy skin
- Fertility

Sources:

Retinol is found in meat, fish, eggs and dairy produce. Beta-carotene is present in brightly coloured fruits and vegetables. One carrot should provide your RDA of vitamin A.

- ●●● liver
- ●●● cod liver oil
- ●●● carrots
- ●● sweet potatoes
- ● butter
- ● tomatoes

Supplements

Multivitamin tablets usually contain at least 800mcg of vitamin A, and intakes of up to 3000mcg of vitamin A per day are considered safe. Because vitamin A is stored in your body it does not need to be taken daily, but it can build up in the liver, and retinol is toxic in high doses. Zinc is required for vitamin A to be released from the liver.

Precautions

Vitamin A as retinol can cause birth defects in an unborn child and should not be taken as a supplement by pregnant women or those planning to become pregnant. Pregnant women should also avoid cod liver oil and liver, as these contain high amounts of retinol. Excessive amounts of beta-carotene turn your skin yellow, but your colour will return to normal if you reduce the dose.

Vitamin B¹ (Thiamin)

Needed to convert carbohydrates into energy and keep your body and mind in good shape, vitamin B¹ is present in many foods but, like all the B vitamins, is easily lost from the body because it is water-soluble.

How it works

Vitamin B¹ is essential for converting food into energy and for the transmission of electrical signals in the nerves and muscles. It also has an important role in the formation of red blood cells and a number of digestive processes.

Known as the 'morale vitamin', thiamin is crucial for the proper functioning of the nervous system and can have a powerful effect on your mood and alertness.

Deficiency symptoms

- Weakness and muscle pains
- Irritability
- Numbness and prickling in legs
- Water retention
- Nausea and stomach pains
- Poor concentration

Remedies

Mind and emotion Probably the main use of vitamin B¹ supplements is for treating mood disorders. Studies have shown that people with a high thiamin intake are less likely to suffer from low self-esteem and depression. It can also help to alleviate sleeping problems.

Concentration and alertness Vitamin B¹ has been found to be beneficial in boosting memory and mental agility, especially in older people.

Alcoholism Vitamin B¹ can help to relieve the symptoms of alcohol withdrawal. It is also needed to replace thiamin that has been lost through alcohol abuse.

Energy booster Vitamin B¹ can increase energy levels and lower blood pressure, improving all-round health.

Thiamin is called the 'morale vitamin' because it helps you to feel positive and happy, and it is now widely used in the treatment of depression and anxiety.

vital facts
Vitamin B^1 (Thiamin)

Recommended daily allowance for adults:

1.4mg

Main functions:

- Converts food into energy
- Keeps the brain functioning well
- Makes you feel good
- Improves all-round health

Sources:

Most foods contain at least a small amount of vitamin B^1, although the more you process food – by chopping or preserving – the more you remove the thiamin. High temperatures also destroy vitamin B^1; by toasting a slice of bread you lose up to a third of its thiamin content.

- ● ● ● whole grains
- ● ● ● brown rice
- ● ● wholemeal pasta
- ● ● pork
- ● ● yeast extract
- ● peas
- ● peanuts
- ● pulses

Supplements

Multivitamin tablets usually contain 1.4mg of vitamin B^1, which is sufficient for an average person to stay healthy and avoid deficiency. People who need to raise their level of alertness or improve their mood can take up to 50mg for medicinal purposes. An increased amount of thiamin is most effective when taken as part of a B-complex supplement.

Vitamin B^1 is easily destroyed by alcohol, caffeine and stress. Pregnant women, smokers, heavy drinkers and those who eat a lot of carbohydrates may need to take a supplement.

Precautions

Although no toxicity has ever been recorded, you should ask your doctor to monitor your intake if you have blood or heart problems. Large amounts can also prevent your body from taking up other B vitamins, so you should avoid taking extra doses.

Vitamin B^2 (Riboflavin)

Helps to convert food into energy by working with enzymes to turn fats, proteins and carbohydrates into a form the cells can use. Deficiency is common: vitamin B^2 is easily destroyed by sunlight and a pint of milk left on the doorstep can lose all its riboflavin within a couple of hours.

How it works

Riboflavin promotes healthy growth and reproductive function, and may help with normal development of the foetus during early pregnancy. Vitamin B^2 is needed to form hair, skin and nails, and for good vision.

Riboflavin has antioxidant qualities and boosts your immune system by helping to form antibodies, blood proteins that seek out and destroy foreign substances. A lack of riboflavin can stop vitamin B^6 from working.

Deficiency symptoms

- Itchy eyes, sensitive to bright lights
- Eczema
- Mouth ulcers, cold sores and cracked lips
- Hair loss

Remedies

Eye problems Vitamin B^2 helps protect against cataracts, benefits vision and eases eye strain.

Concentration and alertness People who have a good intake of vitamin B^2 are more likely to perform well in tests that measure mental functioning.

Female problems Riboflavin helps convert vitamin B^6 into its active form and is usually included in supplements designed to relieve premenstrual syndrome or menopausal disorders.

Cracked, sore lips Vitamin B^2 reduces inflammation of the tongue and lips, and mouth sores.

Essential for energy production, riboflavin helps to boost the immune system and rid your body of toxins.

vital facts
Vitamin B^2 (Riboflavin)

Recommended daily allowance for adults:

1.6mg

Main functions:

- Promotes healthy skin, hair and nails
- Benefits vision
- Helps convert food into energy
- Antioxidant
- Boosts immunity

Sources:

You would need to eat two large bowls of fortified breakfast cereal with skimmed milk to obtain the RDA of riboflavin. Vitamin B^2 dissolves in cooking liquids but is not destroyed by heat. Store foods in a dark place to prevent riboflavin being destroyed by sunlight.

- ● ● ● yeast extract
- ● ● ● whole grains
- ● ● liver
- ● ● fortified breakfast cereals
- ● ● cheese
- ● milk
- ● green, leafy vegetables

Supplements

Multivitamin tablets usually contain 1.6mg of vitamin B^2, which is sufficient for the average person to remain healthy and avoid deficiency. Slightly higher amounts are needed during pregnancy, breastfeeding and during times of stress (including anxiety, overwork, disease and after surgery). Levels of up to 50mg can be taken and even higher doses may be prescribed for conditions such as migraine. Selenium improves absorption from the intestines.

Women taking oral contraceptives, those who exercise regularly, diabetics, vegans, older people and heavy drinkers may need to increase their daily intake of riboflavin.

Precautions

Vitamin B^2 is non-toxic but excess results in bright yellow-green urine. People prone to cataracts should not take more than 10mg of riboflavin daily.

Vitamin B³ (Niacin)

Essential for a healthy nervous system and for the production of sex hormones, vitamin B³ is present in a number of foods and can also be made in your body from an amino acid called tryptophan.

How it works

Like vitamins B¹ and B², niacin is essential for the release of energy from food and the use of oxygen in cells. It helps to maintain healthy skin, nerves, digestive system and brain function. Niacin also helps to balance blood sugar and cholesterol levels, increases circulation and reduces blood pressure, and is thought to protect against some forms of heart disease.

Vitamin B³ takes the form of nicotinic acid, which can cause flushing, and nicotinamide, which does not.

Deficiency symptoms

- Poor memory
- Anxiety or depression
- Headaches
- Fatigue
- Eczema
- Diarrhoea

Remedies

Mind and emotions Studies have shown that people with a low level of niacin are more likely to suffer from depression and poor self-esteem. Niacin therapy is commonly used in cases of acute schizophrenia.

Healthy heart Megadoses of niacin taken under medical supervision have been shown to reduce blood cholesterol. Because it reduces high blood pressure and increases circulation, it is valuable in maintaining a healthy heart.

Digestive problems Niacin helps to keep your digestive system healthy and can ease attacks of diarrhoea.

Niacin is beneficial for a range of health problems and is widely used in the treatment of mental illness.

vital facts
Vitamin B³ (Niacin)

Recommended daily allowance for adults:

18mg

Arthritis Supplements of vitamin B³ have been shown to increase mobility and reduce inflammation.

Alcoholism Niacin supplements can help to reduce alcohol craving and normalize sleeping patterns.

Supplements

Multivitamin tablets usually contain 18mg of vitamin B³, which is sufficient for an average person to avoid deficiency. You only need a slightly higher amount if you exercise a lot, are taking the contraceptive pill or are under stress. Levels of up to 100mg may be beneficial and are best taken as part of a B-complex supplement.

Precautions

High doses of niacin may cause liver malfunction, flushing and headaches. Do not take more than 100mg unless under medical supervision. Pregnant women, people with diabetes and those suffering from liver disorders, stomach ulcers or gout should not take megadoses of vitamin B³.

Main functions:

- Helps maintain mental health
- Releases energy from food
- Promotes proper growth and development
- Good for the heart and circulation

Sources:

Many foods contain vitamin B³ and fortified breakfast cereals are a good source for children. The more food is processed – by chopping, preserving or cooking – the more the niacin content is depleted.

- ●●● lean meat
- ●●● whole grains
- ●●● brewer's yeast
- ●● cheese
- ●● fish
- ● eggs
- ● wholemeal bread

Vitamin B⁵ (Pantothenic acid)

Pantothenic acid has become a popular supplement in recent years because of its ability to boost the immune system, improve energy levels and reduce stress. Present in many foods, vitamin B⁵ is easily destroyed by food processing and preserving, and deficiency is common.

How it works

Like other B vitamins, pantothenic acid is essential for the conversion of food into energy. It is also crucial for the conversion of choline into acetylcholine, a chemical messenger that carries electrical signals between the nerves and muscles and enables your body to function properly.

Vitamin B⁵ is particularly important in controlling the breakdown of fats in your body and may be beneficial during weight-loss diets. It stimulates cell growth, which helps to maintain healthy hair and skin and promote more rapid wound healing.

Deficiency symptoms

- Fatigue
- Anxiety
- Poor concentration
- Tingling hands and feet
- Muscle cramps and tremors
- Headache

Remedies

Stress buster Pantothenic acid reduces stress levels by helping to make anti-stress hormones and controlling the action of the adrenal glands (which go into overdrive during times of stress).

Healthy heart Vitamin B⁵ lowers cholesterol levels and can help to protect against heart disease.

Infection Pantothenic acid is needed to produce antibodies, proteins that destroy foreign substances in the blood, and therefore helps to fight infection.

Hair and skin problems Pantothenic acid is said to prevent hair loss and greying and is often added to shampoos and conditioners. It also helps to rejuvenate skin and heal wounds.

Supplements

Multivitamin tablets usually contain 6mg of vitamin B⁵, which is thought to be adequate for an average person to remain healthy and avoid deficiency.

Vitamin B^5 (Pantothenic acid)

Recommended daily allowance for adults:

6mg

Main functions:

You may need a slightly higher amount as you get older. Levels of up to 300mg can be taken, and it works best as part of a B-complex supplement.

Regular consumption of caffeine and alcohol, smoking, and taking sleeping pills and contraceptives can all deplete vitamin B^5 levels.

- Vital for energy
- Immune system booster
- Keeps skin and hair in good condition
- Reduces stress levels

Precautions

Vitamin B^5 is not known to be toxic, but you should not take doses of more than 300mg per day without medical supervision. Some people experience stomach upsets when taking megadoses.

Pantothenic acid is widely available in foods and in our body tissues; its name comes from the Greek _panthos_, meaning 'everywhere'.

Sources:

Vitamin B^5 is available in many foods, but is easily destroyed by preparing, cooking and preserving (from freezing to canning). Cooking meat reduces the pantothenic acid content by more than a third.

- ● ● ● royal jelly
- ● ● ● brewer's yeast
- ● ● ● liver and kidney
- ● ● nuts
- ● ● whole grains
- ● eggs

Vitamin B⁶ (Pyridoxine)

A group of water-soluble substances that work together and are converted into the active form pyridoxine in your body. Vitamin B⁶ is popular with women who suffer from premenstrual syndrome as it is thought to regulate levels of sex hormones.

How it works

Vitamin B⁶ is essential for the breakdown of food and the production of energy in your body, and it has to be present for vitamin B¹² to be absorbed. It helps to reduce skin inflammation and keeps your teeth and gums healthy.

Pyridoxine is needed to keep the nervous system in good working order and for the formation of antibodies and white blood cells, which fight infection.

Deficiency symptoms

- Water retention
- Anxiety, irritability and depression
- Tingling hands
- Muscle cramps and spasms
- Anaemia

Particularly beneficial for women, pyridoxine can alleviate many symptoms of premenstrual syndrome and the menopause.

Remedies

Female problems Because it helps to balance sex hormones, vitamin B⁶ is widely used to relieve the symptoms of premenstrual syndrome (PMS) and menopause, such as mood swings and depression, and may help in some cases of infertility.

Mind and emotions Vitamin B⁶ is involved in the production of the brain chemicals serotonin and melatonin, which regulate the sleep cycle and have a powerful effect on mood. It is used to treat depression.

Fatigue Vitamin B⁶ increases energy levels and can be beneficial to people with long-term tiredness.

Nausea Vitamin B⁶ alleviates nausea and is included in many remedies for morning sickness.

Acne Pyridoxine helps to balance sex hormones and is used to treat acne.

Recommended daily allowance for adults:

2mg

Main functions:

- Helps to convert food into energy
- Maintains a healthy immune system
- Balances sex hormones and alleviates symptoms of PMS
- Improves low moods

Supplements

About 2mg of vitamin B^6 is sufficient for an average person to remain healthy and avoid deficiency. Slightly higher amounts are needed during pregnancy, breastfeeding and by women who are taking the contraceptive pill or hormone replacement therapy. Heavy drinkers, smokers and those taking antibiotics may need supplements. The more protein you eat, the more vitamin B^6 you need. Vitamin B^6 should always be taken as part of a B-complex supplement and in equal amounts with vitamins B^1 and B^2. You can take up to 100mg, but should seek medical advice before doing so.

Precautions

Prolonged high doses may cause nerve problems such as pins and needles. People with Parkinson's disease who are taking levodopa should not supplement this vitamin.

Sources:

A regular intake of vitamin B^6 is essential, as it is excreted in urine. Pyridoxine is present in many foods, but is easily destroyed by storing, processing and cooking. The RDA can be obtained from a portion of chicken and a baked potato.

- ●●● wheatgerm
- ●●● bananas
- ●● chicken
- ●● fish
- ●● brussels sprouts
- ●● potatoes
- ● wholemeal bread
- ● green, leafy vegetables
- ● baked beans

Vitamin B^{12} (Cobalamin)

Essential for a healthy nervous system, vitamin B^{12} is also needed for growth when we are young and is known to play a part in controlling appetite. Vegans and vegetarians are likely to be deficient in vitamin B^{12} because it is not usually found in plant sources.

How it works

The process of growth requires body cells to divide and multiply constantly. Vitamin B^{12} is needed for cell division and the production of red blood cells. It is also involved in the production of the myelin sheath, a covering that protects nerves and speeds up the passage of electrical impulses along the length of the nerve.

Deficiency symptoms

- Anaemia
- Poor hair condition
- Fatigue
- Eczema or dermatitis
- Tender or sore muscles
- Irritability and anxiety
- Poor memory

Remedies

Fatigue An inadequate intake of vitamin B^{12} causes anaemia, a condition in which a shortage of oxygen-carrying red blood cells results in excessive tiredness. Vitamin B^{12} supplements and injections are prescribed widely by doctors to treat many problems that affect energy levels.

Mood problems Vitamin B^{12} appears to be involved in the production of the brain's feel-good chemicals serotonin and dopamine, which control mood and sleep patterns. An increased intake of vitamin B^{12} may alleviate depression and improve mood.

Healthy blood Pernicious anaemia, the form of anaemia that develops when there is a lack of vitamin B^{12}, can be treated successfully with injections of vitamin B^{12}.

The only vitamin to contain essential minerals, vitamin B^{12} increases energy levels and promotes healthy growth in children.

vital facts
Vitamin B^{12} (Cobalamin)

Recommended daily allowance for adults:

1mcg

Main functions:

- Promotes growth
- Maintains a healthy nervous system
- Prevents anaemia
- Increases energy

Sources:

Vitamin B^{12} is not found in plants but is added to foods as a fortified ingredient. One egg should supply the RDA.

- ● ● ● liver
- ● ● beef
- ● ● pork
- ● ● white fish
- ● ● eggs
- ● fortified breakfast cereal
- ● yeast extract
- ● milk

Supplements

Unlike most water-soluble vitamins, B^{12} can be stored in the liver. Multivitamin tablets usually contain 1mcg of vitamin B^{12}, which is sufficient for an average person to remain healthy and avoid deficiency. Strict vegetarians and vegans will need to take supplements or eat foods fortified with vitamin B^{12}. Women who are pregnant or breastfeeding and older people need slightly higher amounts (the ability to absorb vitamin B^{12} decreases with age). Drinkers, smokers and those taking medicines for stomach ulcers may need more vitamin B^{12}. Levels of up to 100mcg can be taken. Vitamin B^{12} works well with folic acid and is best taken as part of a B-complex supplement.

Precautions

Vitamin B^{12} is not considered to be toxic but there have been rare reports of allergic reaction to injections.

Biotin

A member of the vitamin B group, also known as vitamin H or co-enzyme R, biotin works with other B vitamins to convert food into energy. It is found in many common foods and deficiency is unusual unless you eat a lot of raw egg whites.

How it works

Biotin plays an important part in the production of fatty acids, which are essential for healthy skin, hair and nerves, as well as many other bodily functions. It is thought to help prevent your hair turning grey and to prevent premature baldness.

A regular intake of biotin is essential because it dissolves in water and is excreted in urine.

Deficiency symptoms
- Cradle cap in infants
- Eczema and dermatitis
- Premature greying hair or baldness

Remedies

Hair health Although there is no scientific evidence to support the claim, biotin may help to prevent hair from turning grey and being lost prematurely.

Weight control Because biotin plays a role in fat metabolism it is thought that supplements may aid weight loss.

Healthy skin People who have eczema and/or dermatitis have noted improvements in their skin condition when taking extra biotin. It is also used to treat cradle cap.

Widely used in the treatment of dry skin conditions, biotin is essential for breaking down and metabolizing fats in your body.

vital facts
Biotin

Recommended daily allowance for adults:

150mcg

Main functions:

- Good for hair and skin health
- Alleviates eczema and dermatitis
- May help with weight loss

Sources:

Readily available in many foods in small amounts. If you eat a varied diet, deficiency should not be a problem. Biotin is depleted by alcohol, cooking and refining food, antibiotics and raw egg whites, which contain a protein (avidin) that prevents biotin absorption in the intestines.

- ● ● ● peanuts
- ● ● almonds
- ● ● kidney
- ● ● egg yolk
- ● walnuts
- ● chicken
- ● sesame seeds

Thrush Low levels of biotin are thought to affect your immunity to yeast infections, and high-dose biotin supplements seem to be helpful in alleviating the condition in some people. There are bacteria present in your intestines that produce biotin, but they are easily destroyed by antibiotics. This is why you are more vulnerable to thrush if you are taking antibiotics.

Supplements

A balanced diet should supply the RDA of 150mcg of biotin. Infants with dermatitis and pregnant women may need slightly higher amounts, as will those taking long-term antibiotics (for example as a treatment for acne). Levels of up to 200mcg can be taken, usually as part of a B-complex supplement. Supplements containing biotin are best taken with food.

Precautions

Biotin is non-toxic and no adverse effects have been reported from taking high doses.

Folic acid

A member of the B-complex family, folic acid works with other B vitamins, particularly vitamin B^{12}. Although it is present in many foods, folic acid is easily lost from your body and folic acid deficiency is thought to be the most common vitamin deficiency in the Western world.

How it works
Folic acid is essential for cell division, the production of red blood cells and the metabolism of proteins and sugars. It is involved in the transmission of the genetic code to offspring and is therefore vital during the early stages of pregnancy to ensure the development of a healthy baby.

Deficiency symptoms
- Anaemia
- Cracked lips
- Depression
- Lack of energy
- Poor appetite

Remedies
Birth defects Folic acid is crucial for normal development of the spine and spinal cord during the first three months of pregnancy. Women who intend to become pregnant are advised to take a daily supplement of 400mcg of folic acid before conception and for the first three months of pregnancy to reduce the risk of spina bifida, a congenital condition in which part of the bony spine that helps to protect the spinal cord does not develop properly.

Anaemia Folic acid supplements help to produce healthy red blood cells and thus prevent tiredness and fatigue. However, high amounts of folic acid can hide the symptoms of pernicious anaemia (caused by a lack of vitamin B^{12}) until irreversible brain and nerve damage have occurred.

Essential for the development of a healthy baby, folic acid takes its name from foliage, or green leaves, in which it is often found.

vital facts
Folic acid

Recommended daily allowance for adults:

200mcg

Main functions:

- Prevents some birth defects
- Helps ward off anaemia
- Maintains a healthy body
- May reduce the risk of heart disease

Sources:

Folic acid is found in many foods but it is easily destroyed: up to two-thirds of folic acid is lost in cooking, especially boiling. You need to eat three servings of fortified breakfast cereal to achieve the RDA.

- ● ● ● wheatgerm
- ● ● ● liver
- ● ● ● fortified breakfast cereal
- ● ● ● black-eyed beans
- ● ● green, leafy vegetables (such as spinach and broccoli)
- ● ● peanuts
- ● bananas
- ● avocado

Osteoporosis Folic acid is thought to help maintain strong bones.

Heart problems Folic acid helps to lower levels of the amino acid homocysteine, which is thought to damage the arteries and increase the risk of heart disease.

Supplements

Multivitamin tablets usually contain the RDA of 200mcg of folic acid, which is enough for an average person to remain healthy. Those at risk of folic acid deficiency include heavy drinkers, elderly people and pregnant women, for whom daily supplements of 400–800mcg are recommended.

Precautions

Folic acid is toxic in large doses. It may also cause sleeplessness and interfere with the absorption of zinc in your body. People with epilepsy should consult their doctor before supplementing folic acid as it can interfere with the action of anti-epileptic drugs.

Choline and inositol

These are members of the B-complex family valued for their ability to break down fat and improve memory and brain function. Inositol is not a true vitamin because our bodies can make small amounts of it, but it is normally found in B-complex supplements because it works with choline.

How they work

Choline and inositol help to form lecithin, which helps to break fats into smaller particles that can be used in your body and controls cholesterol build-up. They also help to maintain cell membranes and are important in nourishing brain cells. Choline is used in the production of acetylcholine, a chemical that transmits messages between the nerves and muscles, and is thought to improve memory, mood and athletic performance.

Choline also helps to cleanse your system by enabling the liver to eliminate toxins more effectively.

Deficiency symptoms

- Eczema
- Memory problems
- Nervousness
- High blood pressure
- Frequent coughs and colds

Remedies

Healthy heart and blood vessels Choline and inositol help to break down fat and prevent the build-up of fatty deposits on the walls of your arteries (vessels that carry blood from the heart).

Concentration and alertness Choline in particular has been found to improve memory storage and retrieval, especially in older people.

Choline and inositol help keep your body and mind in good shape by breaking down fat and boosting brain power.

vital facts
Choline and inositol

None established

Weight control By breaking down fat and preventing it from forming deposits, choline and inositol are considered to be valuable slimming aids.

Stress Because of their positive effects on the nervous system, choline and inositol can reduce stress levels and make you feel calmer.

Supplements

Although there is no RDA, most B-complex supplements contain 100mg of choline and inositol. Nutritionists consider a daily intake of between 400 and 1000mg to be beneficial. Heavy drinkers and women taking the contraceptive pill may need higher amounts of both choline and inositol; coffee drinkers need extra inositol.

Precautions

Both choline and inositol are considered safe supplements, but high doses have been thought to worsen depression.

Main functions:

- Lower cholesterol levels
- Weight control
- Boost memory and concentration
- Maintain healthy nervous system

Sources:

Food processing and cooking destroy choline and inositol. A steak or a handful of nuts should supply your daily needs.

- ● ● ● liver
- ● ● ● steak
- ● ● egg yolks
- ● ● brewer's yeast
- ● ● peanuts
- ● citrus fruits
- ● wholemeal bread

Vitamin C (Ascorbic acid)

A powerful antioxidant, vitamin C is also thought to boost immunity and fight a number of diseases. It is water-soluble and quickly lost from your body, so a daily intake is vital.

How it works

Vitamin C is involved in a large number of biological processes, which is why it is essential for health. It is used to make collagen, the protein that makes the skin, joints and bones strong. Vitamin C speeds up wound healing, and helps to form red blood cells and prevent bleeding. Your body's immune system relies on vitamin C to keep the disease-fighting white blood cells active. Vitamin C also helps your body to absorb iron and folic acid effectively and turn food into energy.

Deficiency symptoms

- Bleeding gums
- Easy bruising
- Aches and pains
- Frequent colds and infections
- Red pimples on the skin
- Nosebleeds

Remedies

Colds and flu Vitamin C reduces the duration of colds and other viral infections by killing off viruses and mopping up inflammatory chemicals produced during infection. It also boosts immunity and resistance.

Hay fever As a natural antihistamine, vitamin C helps to reduce the effects of pollen allergy.

Skin care Vitamin C protects against skin damage and reduces the effect of sunburn by neutralizing free radicals and producing collagen.

Fertility Vitamin C is considered essential for sperm health, improving the quality, quantity and mobility of normal sperm. It is also thought to protect genetic material because of its antioxidant qualities.

Wound healing Increasing vitamin C intake helps to speed up the healing process after operations.

Eyesight As an antioxidant, vitamin C protects the eyes from free radical attack, which clouds the lens, and is thought to be particularly important in preventing the development of age-related cataracts.

Osteoporosis Vitamin C is essential for the formation of collagen, which is vital for healthy bones.

vital facts
Vitamin C (Ascorbic acid)

60mg

Supplements

Multivitamin tablets usually contain 60mg of vitamin C, which is necessary for health. Smokers require much more (25mg is lost with every cigarette). Heavy drinkers, those under stress and people who regularly take aspirin or antibiotics or are suffering from infection also need increased amounts. A good basic intake is considered to be 100–250mg daily. Vitamin C works best with calcium and magnesium, and bioflavanoids found in fruits and vegetables enhance its absorption.

Precautions

Megadoses of vitamin C can have a laxative effect, and some people find large doses too acidic (try the low-acid versions instead). If you are taking a megadose, do not stop it suddenly – reduce the amount gradually or you may suffer symptoms of scurvy.

As one of the main antioxidants, vitamin C helps to counteract the effects of free radicals, destructive chemicals that speed up the ageing process and cause cell damage.

Main functions:

- Keeps skin healthy
- Fights infections
- Protects eyesight
- Antioxidant

Sources:

Fresh fruits and vegetables are good sources of vitamin C, and one orange should supply the RDA. Water, cooking, heat and light all destroy vitamin C.

- ● ● ● blackcurrants
- ● ● green pepper
- ● ● mango
- ● ● oranges
- ● ● cabbage
- ● tomatoes
- ● potatoes

Vitamin D

Produced by the body when the skin is exposed to sunlight, and found in foods of animal origin, vitamin D is crucial for the development of healthy bones and teeth, particularly during childhood. Without it, your body cannot build or maintain strong bones.

How it works

Vitamin D is a fat-soluble vitamin that controls calcium absorption, which affects bone development and is also essential for blood clotting. When vitamin D is in short supply, less calcium is absorbed from food and blood levels have to be maintained by taking calcium from bones.

Also known as the 'sunshine vitamin', the body stops producing vitamin D once you have got a suntan.

Deficiency symptoms

- Backache
- Tooth decay
- Twisted limbs in children
- Brittle, painful bones

Remedies

Osteoporosis Elderly people and those at risk of developing osteoporosis may benefit from taking vitamin D supplements to increase calcium absorption and strengthen bones.

Healthy teeth Vitamin D supplements can strengthen teeth and reduce bone loss caused by gum disease.

Rickets Vitamin D prevents the childhood disease rickets, which causes soft, malformed bones.

Psoriasis Some people with psoriasis find that their symptoms improve when they increase their daily intake of vitamin D.

Supplements

If you have plenty of exposure to sunlight you are unlikely to need vitamin D supplements. People who cover themselves up from the sun (for example followers of certain religions), particularly if they are vegetarians or vegans; night workers; those who use

Vitamin D is known as the 'sunshine vitamin' and is essential for healthy bones and teeth.

vital facts
Vitamin D

Recommended daily allowance for adults:

5mcg

Main functions:

- Helps build healthy teeth and bones
- Prevents rickets
- Controls calcium absorption

Sources:

The adult RDA can be obtained from two canned pilchards. Eating fried foods can reduce your body's absorption of vitamin D, as can mineral oil (used in laxatives) and a smoggy atmosphere.

- ● ● ● cod liver oil
- ● ● ● herrings
- ● ● ● mackerel
- ● ● pilchards
- ● ● sardines
- ● salmon
- ● margarine
- ● tuna
- ● cheddar cheese

high-factor sunscreens; and those who are housebound may need to take supplements. Because vitamin D is found mainly in animal products, vegetarians and vegans may need supplements. Pregnant and breastfeeding women may also benefit from vitamin D supplements. Multivitamin tablets usually contain 5mcg of vitamin D, but you may need twice this amount if you are over 50. You should not take more than five times the RDA.

Precautions

Vitamin D is the most toxic vitamin and side effects include vomiting, headaches, diarrhoea and depression. Taking cod liver oil and vitamin D supplements can result in excessive intake. Children are most at risk of overdosing on vitamin D and should not be given supplements unless under strict medical supervision.

Vitamin E (Tocopherol)

A key antioxidant, vitamin E is particularly important for a healthy heart and blood supply and is very good for your skin. Although it is fat-soluble, this vitamin is only stored in your body for a short period of time and regular intake is essential.

How it works

Vitamin E is a powerful antioxidant that helps to protect your body from the effects of free radicals, which damage cells and speed up the ageing process. One of its key functions is as an anticoagulant: it reduces abnormal blood clotting and helps keep blood vessels free from blockages. It is therefore considered crucial in protecting against heart and blood vessel disease.

Vitamin E is important for the production of energy from food and the maintenance of health at every level. It helps to control body temperature and is used to treat hot flushes that can occur during menopause. Vitamin E also helps to improve the activity of vitamin A in your body.

Deficiency symptoms

- Easy bruising
- Slow wound healing
- Lack of sex drive
- Exhaustion after exercise
- Varicose veins

Remedies

Infections Vitamin E is thought to boost the immune system and help your body to fight infection.

Heart and circulation Studies have shown that vitamin E can help to keep your heart and blood vessels healthy. It is also used to alleviate varicose veins.

Healthy skin Vitamin E speeds up wound healing and prevents thick scar formation. Its antioxidant effects help keep your skin looking young and in good condition.

Eye problems Supplements of vitamin E are thought to prevent cataract formation and eyesight loss with age.

Infertility Vitamin E, sometimes known as the 'anti-sterility vitamin', is thought to be particularly helpful in cases of male infertility as it increases the amount of sperm produced.

vital facts
Vitamin E (Tocopherol)

Recommended daily allowance for adults:

10mg

Main functions:

- Antioxidant
- Keeps your skin looking young
- Important for fertility
- Reduces the symptoms of menopause
- Maintains a healthy blood supply

Sources:

Vitamin E is present in many foods, and a handful of sunflower seeds should supply the RDA. Heating destroys a third of a food's vitamin E content and freezing destroys up to 80 per cent.

- ●●● wheatgerm oil
- ●●● sunflower oil
- ●●● sunflower seeds
- ●● almonds
- ●● pine nuts
- ●● peanut butter
- ●● sweet potato
- ● asparagus
- ● spinach
- ● avocado

Supplements

Vitamin E deficiency is unusual, as it is found in many foods. Multivitamin tablets usually contain 10mg of vitamin E, but doses of up to 1000mg are considered safe to take under medical supervision. Pregnant or breastfeeding women, and women taking the contraceptive pill or going through menopause may benefit from increased amounts of vitamin E. Those suffering from heart or blood vessel problems may need to take supplements. Vitamin E works best with vitamin C and selenium, and absorption is reduced by high intakes of iron.

Precautions

If you are taking medicines to thin the blood, or have diabetes, consult your doctor before taking vitamin E supplements. High doses should only be taken under medical guidance.

One of the main antioxidant vitamins, vitamin E's key function is its role in maintaining a healthy blood supply.

Calcium

Your body contains more calcium than any other mineral. Best known for giving us strong bones and teeth, calcium is essential for a whole range of body processes. Many people are at risk of calcium deficiency, particularly women and elderly people.

How it works

About 99 per cent of calcium from your diet goes straight to your teeth and bones, where it is used for building and maintaining strength. The other 1 per cent is used throughout your body to help muscles contract, enable blood to clot, transmit messages along nerves, produce energy, and keep your heart beating and your immune system in tiptop condition. Because calcium plays such an important role in so many processes, if stores are low your body takes what it needs from your bones, causing the bones to become thin and brittle. A good intake of calcium is therefore essential throughout life, particularly during childhood and adolescence, when bones are growing, and during old age, when bones become thinner and more brittle.

Deficiency symptoms

- Sleeplessness
- Muscle cramps or twitching
- Arthritis or other joint pain
- Tooth decay
- High blood pressure

Remedies

Osteoporosis Supplements have been shown to help slow down bone loss in older women, reducing the risk of osteoporosis and bone fractures. Calcium helps to treat the condition once it exists.

Cramp and period pains Calcium supplements may help to relieve leg cramps, including those associated with pregnancy. Increased amounts may ease period pains.

Depression, panic attacks and insomnia Calcium is used to treat a range of mood disorders and can also help sleeping problems.

High blood pressure Calcium is thought to protect against the development of high blood pressure, particularly during pregnancy.

Tooth loss Most teeth are lost through periodontal disease, which causes loss of jaw bone. Calcium supplements help to prevent and treat this.

vital facts
Calcium

Recommended daily allowance for adults:

800mg

Main functions:

- Maximizes bone density
- Keeps your heartbeat regular
- Maintains your immune system
- Reduces the risk of osteoporosis

Sources:

A pint of semi-skimmed milk should provide an adequate daily intake of calcium. Chocolate, rhubarb, spinach and bran contain substances that interfere with calcium absorption.

- ●●● semi-skimmed or skimmed milk
- ●●● cheddar cheese
- ●● sardines
- ●● tofu
- ●● dried figs
- ●● watercress
- ●● yogurt
- ● cabbage
- ● eggs

Supplements

Calcium depends on vitamin D for its effective absorption, and works with magnesium and phosphorus.

The recommended range of calcium intake is 800–1200mg daily, although it is safe to take higher amounts because any excess is excreted in urine. Those on low-fat diets, vegans, pregnant or breastfeeding women and older women may need supplements.

Precautions

Very high doses of calcium might cause kidney stones and interfere with the absorption of other minerals.

Essential for healthy teeth and bones, calcium is also crucial for conducting messages along nerves and enabling muscles to contract.

Chromium

Helps to control blood sugar levels, reduces hunger pangs and food cravings, and plays a part in the breakdown of fats. As we get older we store less chromium in our bodies and deficiency is thought to be common.

How it works

Chromium is involved in the production of energy from fats and carbohydrates. It seems to work with the hormone insulin to control sugar levels in your body and lower cholesterol levels, and is therefore thought to play a part in preventing the development of diabetes and help with weight loss. It is also thought to help prevent and reduce high blood pressure.

Deficiency symptoms

- Drowsiness
- Need for frequent meals
- Dizziness and irritability after six hours without food
- Craving for sweet foods
- Excessive thirst
- Hot or cold sweats

Remedies

Weight control Supplements may help people to lose weight as chromium has a beneficial effect on fat metabolism, hunger pangs and food cravings.

Blood sugar levels Studies have shown that people who suffer from low blood sugar (hypoglycaemia), which causes anxiety and sweating, have benefited from increasing their intake of chromium. Limited research indicates that people with diabetes may be able to control their blood sugar levels with chromium supplements.

Important for controlling blood sugars, chromium is also popular in weight-control supplements because of its effects on appetite and hunger pangs.

vital facts
Chromium

Main functions:

- Controls blood sugar levels
- May help weight control
- Helps to regulate blood pressure
- Controls cholesterol levels

Sources:

Diets high in sugar are thought to increase the excretion of chromium in urine. Brewer's yeast is the best source of chromium because it contains a form that your body can use much more easily than that obtained from other foods.

- ●●● brewer's yeast
- ●●● egg yolk
- ●● meat
- ●● cheese
- ●● wholemeal bread
- ●● whole grains
- ● spinach
- ● bananas

Healthy heart Chromium supplements may help to lower cholesterol levels, thus reducing the risk of developing heart disease. Chromium also helps to reduce high blood pressure.

Supplements

There is no RDA for chromium but 25mcg a day is thought to be adequate. Supplements containing up to 200mcg are thought to be safe. Older people, those who exercise a lot, people who tend to gain weight and those who eat a lot of processed food may benefit from supplements.

Precautions

Chromium is toxic only if more than 1g a day is taken.

Copper

An essential trace mineral needed for a wide variety of functions in your body. As an antioxidant, copper helps to protect your body from cell damage and ageing, and is widely valued for its ability to reduce the pain and inflammation of arthritis.

How it works

Copper is important for collagen production, which is essential for healthy bones and skin. It plays a role in respiration, by converting iron into the blood's oxygen-carrying pigment haemoglobin. It also plays a part in the action of various proteins needed for growth, is important for proper nerve function and boosts the immune system. It is involved in the production of the pigment melanin, which affects the colour of your skin and hair.

Your body needs copper to be able to use vitamin C effectively. Copper poisons sperm and is therefore used in contraceptive devices such as the coil.

Deficiency symptoms
- Tiredness
- Changes in skin colour
- Anaemia
- Pale skin and diarrhoea in babies
- Loss of sense of taste

Remedies

Arthritis Copper reduces swelling and inflammation and increases joint mobility in those who suffer from arthritis. If you wear a copper bracelet, traces of the mineral are absorbed through the skin into the bloodstream.

Immune system booster Copper increases the white blood cell count, vital for fighting infection.

Best known for relieving the pain and inflammation of arthritis, copper is involved in a number of essential body functions.

vital facts
Copper

None established

Healthy heart and blood vessels Copper is involved in regulating blood cholesterol levels and a low intake of copper is thought to be a contributory factor in heart and circulatory diseases.

Energy booster By helping your body to absorb iron, copper helps to keep up your energy levels.

Supplements
Copper deficiency is rare and there is no RDA for this mineral. Multimineral supplements usually contain 1–2mg of copper, which is sufficient for an average person to remain healthy and avoid deficiency. Elderly people, vegetarians and those taking zinc supplements may need small amounts of extra copper.

Precautions
Excess copper can cause headaches, hair loss, sleeplessness and depression.

Main functions:

- Boosts the immune system
- Relieves symptoms of arthritis
- May protect your heart and blood vessels
- Antioxidant

Sources:

Present in a wide variety of foods, up to 70 per cent of copper is lost when food is processed. A can of sardines or a handful of sunflower seeds should meet your daily needs.

- ● ● ● oysters
- ● ● ● liver
- ● ● ● shellfish
- ● ● ● sardines
- ● ● sunflower seeds
- ● ● peanuts
- ● mushrooms
- ● wholemeal bread
- ● prunes

Iodine

This purple-coloured mineral takes its name from the Greek word *iodes*, meaning 'violet-like'. Iodine is essential for the production of thyroid hormones, which control your energy levels and the rate you burn up fat. It also crucial for a child's physical and intellectual development.

How it works

Iodine is needed to make thyroid hormones, which control your body's metabolic rate, including the speed at which you burn up calories. It plays a major part in preventing tiredness and weight gain, and is included in many slimming products.

Iodine is important in promoting normal growth and mental function. Lack of iodine during pregnancy is a major problem in many parts of the world and can severely affect a baby's brain function and development.

Deficiency symptoms

- Swollen thyroid gland in your neck
- Tiredness
- Breast pain
- Concentration and memory problems
- Cold hands and feet

Remedies

Weight problems Iodine supplements may help to improve the action of a sluggish thyroid gland and help you burn off excess fat.

Painful breasts Studies have shown that increasing iodine intake can reduce the pain and swelling associated with benign (non-cancerous) breast lumps.

Swollen thyroid gland This is a symptom of thyroid deficiency and iodine supplements can help to reduce the swelling (severe cases will require medical treatment).

Energy booster Iodine can improve all-round energy, making you feel better mentally and physically.

With its vital role in determining the rate at which your body burns up calories, iodine is a popular addition to slimming pills.

vital facts
Iodine

Recommended daily allowance for adults:

150mcg

Main functions:

- Healthy growth and development
- Helps control metabolic rate
- Useful in weight-loss programmes
- Relieves tiredness and fatigue

Sources:

Most table salt is fortified with iodine. You can get your daily requirement of this mineral by eating 100g of mackerel.

- ● ● ● kelp (seaweed)
- ● ● ● mackerel and haddock
- ● ● ● mussels
- ● ● canned salmon
- ● ● prawns
- ● milk
- ● onions

Supplements

Vegans may be at risk of slight iodine deficiency, and if you exercise a lot you may need to take supplements because iodine is lost in sweat. Eating large amounts of vegetables of the Cruciferae family, such as cabbage, cauliflower and turnips, prevents iodine absorption. Iodine needs selenium and vitamin A in order to be effective. Multimineral tablets usually contain 150mcg of iodine, which is sufficient for an average person to and avoid deficiency.

Precautions

High doses of iodine are toxic. They may cause acne or make it worse, and can interfere with the action of other hormones in your body. Although amounts of up to 500mcg are considered safe, seek medical advice if you intend to take more than the RDA.

Iron

Essential for life, iron is a component of haemoglobin, the red pigment in blood that transports oxygen to the cells and removes the waste product carbon dioxide. Women are most at risk of iron deficiency because of blood loss through monthly periods.

How it works

Iron is a vital component of red blood cells. It is also needed for the production and release of energy in your body. Iron plays an essential role in maintaining a healthy immune system and helps to destroy invading micro-organisms such as viruses and bacteria.

Iron requirements are thought to double during pregnancy, because the mother produces more red blood cells to supply the growing foetus with oxygen and nourishment.

Deficiency symptoms

- Pale skin
- White or brittle fingernails
- Tiredness
- Sleeplessness
- Loss of appetite
- Itchiness
- Frequent illnesses

Remedies

Iron-deficiency anaemia Iron supplements prevent and cure this disorder.

Painful periods Research suggests that daily iron supplements may alleviate period pains.

Boosts energy levels An increased intake of iron can reduce tiredness and fatigue associated with iron deficiency.

Concentration Studies indicate that iron supplements of the RDA may prevent learning problems and improve children's academic performance.

Essential for the formation of red blood cells, iron improves your energy levels and boosts concentration.

vital facts
iron

Recommended daily allowance for adults:

14mg

Main Functions:

- Boosts energy and reduces fatigue
- Essential for healthy blood
- Strengthens the immune system
- Healthy growth and development

Sources:

A bowl of fortified breakfast cereal such as branflakes will supply the RDA of iron. Avoid drinking tea with meals as this interferes with iron absorption. Boiling vegetables can reduce the iron content by 20 per cent.

- ●●● fortified breakfast cereal
- ●●● liver
- ●● dried fruit
- ●● sardines
- ● canned tuna
- ● parsley
- ● watercress

Supplements

Iron is best taken as part of a multivitamin/multimineral supplement, and the maximum dosage is around 15mg daily, unless under medical supervision. Women are likely to benefit from iron supplements, particularly if pre-menopausal, pregnant, breastfeeding or if pregnancies are close together. Coffee and tea drinkers, athletes, vegetarians and vegans may need to increase their intake of iron.

Iron can only be used to make haemoglobin in the presence of copper. Vitamin C improves the absorption of iron, so drink a glass of orange juice when taking iron supplements.

Precautions

Iron supplements can cause constipation and indigestion. High doses can kill, and it is essential to keep iron tablets out of the reach of children, as only a few pills can be fatal. Consult your doctor before giving your child iron supplements.

Magnesium

A mineral that is essential for every biochemical process that takes place, a shortfall of magnesium will affect just about every part of your body. Deficiency is common, and if you take large amounts of calcium this will hinder magnesium absorption.

How it works

Magnesium is vital for turning food into energy, and also plays a part in the release of the hormone insulin, which regulates blood sugar levels. The nervous system relies on magnesium to function properly and it is valued for its stress-relieving properties.

Magnesium helps to repair and maintain body cells, and is thought to help keep your heart and blood vessels healthy. Because it controls the movement of calcium in and out of cells, magnesium is important for strong bones and teeth. Magnesium also helps to relax muscles.

Deficiency symptoms

- Stress and irritability
- Irregular heartbeat
- Cramp or twitching muscles
- Sleeplessness
- Fatigue
- Depression

Remedies

Premenstrual syndrome Studies indicate that magnesium supplements are extremely effective in reducing the symptoms of premenstrual syndrome (PMS), including alleviating fatigue, irritability, fluid retention and tender breasts. Magnesium may also relieve period pains because of its effects on muscles and nerves.

Depression and mood problems This anti-stress mineral is considered to be very helpful in fighting depression and stabilizing moods, because it is involved in the production of brain chemicals that make you feel good.

This versatile mineral is crucial for numerous functions in your body, including energy production and the synthesis of genetic material.

vital facts
Magnesium

Healthy heart Magnesium helps maintain a healthy cardiovascular system and is thought to ward off heart attacks.

Fatigue An all-round energy booster, magnesium can increase your vitality.

Indigestion Magnesium neutralizes stomach acids, which can cause severe discomfort.

Supplements
Because many people's diets are thought to be deficient in magnesium, supplements of the RDA (300mg) are recommended. Women and heavy drinkers may benefit from extra amounts of magnesium.

Precautions
High amounts of magnesium (1000mg) can be toxic. If you have kidney problems, consult your doctor before supplementing.

Recommended daily allowance for adults:

300mg

Main functions:

- Essential for energy
- Crucial for muscles and nerves
- Keeps bones and teeth strong
- Helps fight depression

Sources:

Magnesium works best with calcium, phosphorus, zinc, and vitamins C and D, while protein foods such as chicken or fish increase its absorption. Substances known as oxalates (found in chocolate, rhubarb and spinach) hinder magnesium absorption. Four slices of wholemeal bread should supply the RDA.

- ●●● nuts
- ●●● wholemeal bread
- ●●● peanut butter
- ●● popcorn
- ●● cheddar cheese
- ●● white fish
- ● eggs
- ● milk

Manganese

A trace mineral that maintains the healthy functioning of the nervous system, manganese is essential for normal brain function, and is used in the treatment of many nervous system disorders. It is also needed for normal growth and development.

How it works

Manganese is important for healthy bones and nerves, is needed for the production of sex hormones and is involved in the production of thyroid hormones, which control the rate at which your body burns up calories. It helps to stabilize blood sugar levels and is needed to make red blood cells, which carry oxygen and nutrients to all cells.

Manganese is needed for the proper breakdown and use of food in your body. It also acts as an antioxidant by activating an enzyme that breaks down potentially harmful free radicals.

Deficiency symptoms

- Poor memory
- Skin rashes
- Twitching muscles
- Painful joints
- Dizziness

Remedies

Osteoporosis Increasing your intake of manganese is thought to strengthen your bones and reduce the risk of developing osteoporosis, a condition that makes bones brittle and liable to fracture.

Wound healing Manganese is needed for the formation of collagen, the connective tissue that gives skin its elasticity, and is thought to speed up wound healing.

Manganese is an important nutrient that is essential for brain function and has a powerful effect on mood.

Mind and emotions Because of its beneficial effects on the nervous system, manganese supplements are widely used to treat depression and other nervous system disorders.

Infertility Manganese is essential for reproduction because it is involved in the production of sex hormones. Supplements may improve fertility, particularly in women.

Supplements

As yet there is no RDA for manganese, but most multimineral preparations contain a small amount and doses up to 5mg daily are considered to be safe, with the optimum level at least 1.4mg daily. Heavy drinkers and those on antibiotics may benefit from increased intake. Zinc, and vitamins B¹, C, E and K are thought to improve its absorption.

Precautions

Manganese is not thought to be toxic, unless it is inhaled (in the form of manganese dust). High doses of manganese may cause learning difficulties in children.

vital facts
Manganese

Recommended daily allowance for adults:

None established

Main functions:

- Vital for brain function
- Improves bone strength
- Helps clean out your system
- Promotes wound healing

Sources:

Large amounts of calcium and phosphorus interfere with the absorption of manganese. A cup of tea should give a sufficient daily intake.

- ● ● ● tea
- ● ● ● wholemeal bread
- ● ● ● avocado
- ● ● ● hazelnuts
- ● ● almonds
- ● ● coconut
- ● plums
- ● bananas
- ● watercress

Molybdenum

Required for optimum health, the functions of molybdenum include helping to make uric acid, a waste product found in urine, and to enable your body to use iron. A lack of molybdenum is thought to contribute to impotence in older men.

How it works

Molybdenum helps your body to make certain enzymes so it can use the energy released from fats and carbohydrates. It also promotes the formation of healthy red blood cells, and is needed to keep nerves healthy.

Molybdenum is thought to be an antioxidant and helps your body to break down harmful substances such as alcohol and sulphites, which are used to preserve food.

Deficiency symptoms

The following are possible symptoms of molybdenum deficiency:

- Anaemia
- Tooth decay
- Impotence
- Irritability
- Poor general health

Remedies

Anaemia By enabling your body to use iron, molybdenum can help prevent some forms of anaemia.

Tooth decay A lack of molybdenum is thought to be a cause of tooth decay.

Mind and emotions Molybdenum is known to promote a feeling of wellbeing and can help you feel more alert.

Sexual problems Molybdenum is considered to be useful in cases of impotence in older men.

Allergies Studies indicate that increasing your intake of molybdenum under medical supervision can relieve the symptoms of allergy and reduce wheezing in asthmatics.

Molybdenum is thought to improve all-round health, keeping your body and mind in good shape.

vital facts
Molybdenum

Recommended daily allowance for adults:

None established

Main functions:

- May reduce allergic symptoms
- Antioxidant
- Energy booster

Sources:

Whole grains, lentils and dark green, leafy vegetables are the best sources of molybdenum. A serving of green beans should meet your nutritional requirements.

- ●●● liver
- ●●● lentils
- ●●● wheatgerm
- ●● sunflower seeds
- ●● green beans
- ●● spinach
- ● eggs
- ● rice
- ● chicken

Supplements

There is no RDA for molybdenum but multivitamin/multimineral tablets may contain 25mcg, which is thought to be sufficient for an average person to avoid deficiency. Extra supplementation is not generally recommended.

Precautions

Do not take extra doses of molybdenum except on the advice of your doctor. Molybdenum makes your body get rid of copper and can cause gout (a build-up of uric acid around the joints).

Phosphorus

Essential for the structure and function of your body, phosphorus is also vital for communication between cells and for energy production. It is found in most foods and deficiency is rare, but too much phosphorus can upset your mineral balance and decrease calcium levels.

How it works

Phosphorus is needed for the production of energy from food and to activate the B-complex vitamins (also involved in energy production). It is a component of genetic material, essential for growth and repair, and combines with calcium to form calcium phosphate, which makes teeth and bones rigid.

Phosphorus requires vitamin D and calcium in order to function and you need to have twice as much calcium as phosphorus for both to work properly.

Deficiency symptoms

- Bone pain
- Weak, soft bones
- Twitching muscles
- Loss of appetite
- Fatigue

Remedies

Bone health Phosphorus is needed to maintain bone density, and an increased intake may shorten the time broken bones take to heal.

Energy booster Phosphorus is valued by athletes because it increases endurance and reduces tiredness.

Essential for the structure and efficiency of your body, phosphorus helps to boost energy levels and fight fatigue.

vital facts
Phosphorus

Recommended daily allowance for adults:

800mg

Main functions:

- Reduces tiredness and increases endurance
- Needed for energy production
- Maintains healthy bones and teeth
- Needed for growth and repair

Alcoholism Phosphorus supplements are thought to reduce alcohol withdrawal symptoms. Heavy drinkers are usually deficient in phosphorus and may need to take a supplement.

Kidney stones Phosphorus reduces the level of calcium in urine and may help to protect against the formation of kidney stones.

Supplements

Multimineral tablets usually include a low dose of phosphorus, despite the fact that deficiency is rare. Antacids and alcohol may interfere with phosphorus levels, and pregnant or breastfeeding women may need slightly higher doses.

Precautions

Fizzy cola drinks may upset your calcium-phosphorus balance (they contain high amounts of phosphotic acid). Extra phosphorus should only be taken under medical supervision.

Sources:

Found in most foods; a pint of semi-skimmed or skimmed milk and a cheese sandwich should provide the RDA.

- ●●● hard cheese
- ●●● milk products
- ●●● yeast
- ●● whole grains
- ●● shellfish
- ●● nuts
- ●● seeds
- ● eggs

Potassium

Your body needs potassium to work properly: it helps muscles to contract, is involved in nerve function, regulates the heartbeat, transfers nutrients to cells and, most important of all, controls the amount of water in body cells.

How it works

Potassium allows nutrients to move into body cells and waste products to move out. It helps to control the production of the hormone insulin, which regulates blood sugar levels, and to maintain normal blood pressure.

Potassium helps the digestive system to function properly, to eliminate waste products and ensures that fluid levels are correctly balanced in your body.

Deficiency symptoms
- Vomiting and diarrhoea
- Muscular weakness
- Low blood pressure
- Extreme thirst
- Swollen abdomen
- Confusion and irritability

Remedies

Mind and emotions By helping to send oxygen to the brain, potassium promotes clear thinking and can relieve symptoms of depression.

Blood pressure Supplements of potassium have been shown to reduce high blood pressure and may help to protect against the risk of stroke.

Cramp Increasing your intake of potassium can relieve muscular cramps.

Energy booster Because it is involved in energy production and muscle contraction, maintaining your potassium level can increase energy levels, improve athletic performance and reduce fatigue.

Essential for maintaining your body's water balance, a good intake of potassium helps to lower raised blood pressure and reduce the risk of stroke.

vital facts
Potassium

Recommended daily allowance for adults:
None established

Supplements

There is no RDA for potassium but it is found in most multivitamin and multimineral supplements and daily intakes of about 3000mg are recommended. If you exercise a lot, live in a hot climate, take diuretics (pills to reduce water retention) or laxatives, are on a low-carbohydrate diet, drink a lot of alcohol or have had a prolonged bout of vomiting and diarrhoea, you may need to increase your intake of potassium. Too much salt in your diet affects potassium levels. Potassium works best with zinc and magnesium.

Precautions

If you have kidney problems or are taking drugs to reduce high blood pressure do not take potassium supplements without seeking advice from your doctor first.

Main functions:

- ● Beats fatigue
- ● Normalizes blood pressure
- ● Maintains water balance within cells
- ● Activates enzymes that control energy production in the body

Sources:

Potassium is found in a wide range of foods and deficiency is only likely if you do not eat many fruits or vegetables. Two bananas a day should supply all the potassium you need.

- ● ● ● bananas
- ● ● ● tomato purée
- ● ● ● spinach
- ● ● cauliflower
- ● ● red pepper
- ● ● potato crisps
- ● ● chicken
- ● oranges
- ● cheddar cheese
- ● red wine

Selenium

A powerful antioxidant, selenium works synergistically with vitamin E, meaning that both are more powerful if taken together. Selenium is necessary for metabolism, helps the liver to work effectively and is present in sperm. Deficiency can be linked to male infertility.

How it works

Selenium helps to activate antioxidant enzymes such as glutathione peroxidase, which neutralizes potentially harmful free radicals, and is therefore important in helping to protect your body from a wide range of diseases. Selenium is needed for healthy muscles, including those in your heart. It also boosts the immune system, increasing your ability to fight infection.

Selenium is needed for good eyesight, it helps to maintain skin and hair health, and is thought to help treat dandruff. It reduces inflammation and relieves many symptoms of menopause.

Essential for sperm production, selenium plays a vital role in maintaining male fertility and sex drive.

Deficiency symptoms

- Frequent infections
- High blood pressure
- Age spots and premature skin wrinkling
- Infertility
- Cataracts
- Dandruff

Remedies

Infections Selenium improves immune system function by increasing the production of the white blood cells that fight infections.

Menopause Selenium supplements can alleviate the symptoms of menopause, including hot flushes.

Hair, skin and nails Selenium improves the condition of hair, skin and nails, helps to reduce scalp flaking and helps maintain your skin's elasticity. It is also thought to help improve acne.

Arthritis Selenium is a useful treatment because it reduces inflammation.

vital facts
Selenium

Main functions:

- Component of male sperm
- Helps to maintain skin elasticity
- Powerful antioxidant
- Stimulates the immune system

Infertility Selenium has a role in male sex drive and is needed for sperm production. Studies indicate that taking selenium supplements increases the chances of conception in cases of male subfertility.

Supplements

There is no RDA as yet for selenium but it has been suggested that an intake of 75mcg daily should be sufficient for an average person to remain healthy and avoid deficiency. Take vitamin E with selenium to ensure maximum benefit of both. Elderly people, smokers, vegetarians and vegans, and pregnant or breastfeeding women may need slightly higher amounts.

Precautions

Selenium is toxic in very small doses. Take no more than 200mg daily unless under medical supervision.

Sources:

A few brazil nuts or a serving of tuna should contain all the selenium your body needs.

- ●●● brazil nuts
- ●●● fish and shellfish
- ●● sunflower seeds
- ●● wholemeal bread
- ●● walnuts
- ● dairy products
- ● fruit and vegetables

Sodium

Crucial for normal growth, sodium enables your muscles and nerves to function properly and helps move nutrients into cells. Like potassium, it is essential for maintaining your body's water balance. Deficiency is unlikely because sodium (as salt) is present in a wide range of foods.

How it works

To function properly, your body needs to have the right balance of potassium and sodium; most of the potassium is in the cells and most of the sodium is in the fluid that bathes them. Between them, they control water balance, make sure body fluids are neither too alkaline nor too acidic, and prevent dehydration.

Like potassium, sodium helps muscles and nerves to function properly.

Deficiency symptoms

- Low blood pressure
- Muscle cramps
- Dizziness
- Loss of appetite
- Headache

Remedies

Rehydration Isotonic drinks contain balanced amounts of potassium, sodium, glucose and water. They should be used to replace fluids and return the concentration of salts and glucose in the blood to normal as quickly as possible following prolonged bouts of sickness or diarrhoea. Babies and young children are particularly vulnerable to dehydration because any water lost accounts for a higher proportion of the total water content in their bodies, and dehydration can occur very quickly. Athletes also use fluid replacement drinks during and after exercise.

Muscle cramps Small increases of sodium may help to alleviate night-time muscle cramps.

Crucial for maintaining your body's water balance and enabling nerves and muscles to function, sodium can also cause serious health problems if taken in excess.

vital facts
Sodium

Eye health Eye drops contain sodium to make them as similar as possible to human tears.

Supplements

The RDA for sodium is 1600mg daily, but average intake is at least twice this amount. Supplements used in cases of heat exhaustion, cramp or following vomiting and/or diarrhoea should only be taken under medical supervision.

Precautions

Too much salt in the diet is linked to high blood pressure and also causes the loss of potassium, which leads to fluid retention. If you have raised blood pressure you should try to decrease the amount of salt in your diet; this can be achieved easily by not adding it during cooking or at the table. Read the labels of processed foods to see how much salt they contain.

Recommended daily allowance for adults:

1600mg

Main functions:

- Maintains your body's water balance
- Important for nerve and muscle function
- Essential for life

Sources:

Sodium, or salt, is present in most foods. A rasher of bacon should provide sufficient sodium for your daily needs.

- ● ● ● table salt
- ● ● ● bacon
- ● ● ● olives
- ● ● ● prawns
- ● ● celery
- ● ● cottage cheese
- ● ● watercress
- ● ● cornflakes
- ● wholemeal bread

Zinc

Needed for enzyme activity essential for your body's normal function and development, zinc also plays a crucial role in the protection and repair of DNA and helps to regulate hormone levels. Most zinc is lost when food is processed, and a lack of zinc is linked to poor growth and infertility.

How it works

Vital for growth and wound healing, zinc is also a powerful antioxidant and immune system booster, helping to protect you from infection. It is also thought to be important for brain function and a healthy nervous system, and is important for mental alertness.

Zinc is crucial for healthy reproductive organs in both men and women. It is needed for the production of healthy sperm, helps form genetic material and is crucial for the development of a healthy foetus. It also helps to maintain your senses of sight, taste and smell.

Deficiency symptoms
- Frequent infections
- Poor wound healing
- Loss of sense of taste and/or smell
- Eczema, acne or psoriasis
- White flecks in the fingernails
- Poor appetite
- Slow nail and hair growth

Remedies

Colds and flu As one of the main protectors of your immune system, zinc is important to help fight infection. In tests, sucking zinc lozenges reduced the length and severity of illnesses such as colds and flu significantly.

Healthy skin Zinc reduces inflammation, and supplements are beneficial for treating acne and other skin complaints such as eczema. Extra zinc speeds up wound healing.

Arthritis As an antioxidant and immune system booster, zinc can help to reduce pain and inflammation.

Infertility Women with irregular periods may benefit from zinc supplements. Zinc is useful in cases of male subfertility because it is important for healthy sperm production and increases potency and sex drive.

vital facts
Zinc

Zinc is crucial for reproduction: it helps make healthy sperm and is needed to form genetic material.

15mg

Main functions:

- Improves wound healing
- Essential for sexual health and fertility
- Necessary for growth and development
- Mainstay of the immune system

Supplements

Multivitamin and multimineral supplements contain varying amounts of zinc. Pregnant women need to increase their intake of zinc slightly to ensure the foetus develops properly. If you are suffering from a cold or infection or have had surgery you may benefit from zinc supplementation. Vegans, vegetarians, women taking oral contraceptives and heavy drinkers may be deficient in zinc. If you are taking high amounts of vitamin B^6 you will need to increase your intake of zinc. The suggested safe upper limit for long-term use is 15mg – the RDA.

Sources:

A single oyster or an 250g (8oz) steak supplies sufficient zinc to meet the RDA.

- ● ● ● oysters
- ● ● steak
- ● ● wheatgerm
- ● ● pumpkin seeds
- ● ● brazil nuts
- ● egg yolk

Precautions

High doses of zinc interfere with the production of healthy blood cells. Amounts up to 50mg are thought to be safe for short-term use but you should consult your doctor first.

Omega-3 oils

Members of the omega-3 fat family, mainly derived from oily fish such as mackerel, salmon and herring, are essential for protecting the nervous system and brain, and are crucial for early development. They have a powerful effect on learning and intelligence and can have a strong influence on your mood.

How they work

Omega-3 fats are used to make cell membranes, sex hormones and hormone-like chemicals known as series 3 prostaglandins. These perform a wide variety of functions in your body: they help to thin the blood and break down blood clots, and also reduce the amount of harmful fats in the blood, which contribute to the risk of heart attacks. They improve immune system function by reducing inflammation, and help to maintain your body's water balance.

These fats are crucial for a baby's brain development during pregnancy.

Deficiency symptoms

- Dry skin
- Frequent infections
- Poor co-ordination
- Memory and concentration problems
- High blood pressure
- Inflammatory diseases such as rheumatoid arthritis, eczema and psoriasis

Remedies

Psoriasis Increasing your intake of oily fish or taking omega-3 supplements has been shown to improve psoriasis in many cases.

Learning difficulties Studies of children suffering from dyslexia and hyperactivity have indicated that they benefit from supplements containing omega-3 oils.

Weight loss Increasing your intake of omega-3 oils may help you to reduce body fat by removing fat from fat cells and transporting it to muscle tissue where it is converted into energy.

Heart disease Omega-3 fats benefit your heart by reducing the amount of harmful fats and improving blood flow. They also appear to lower the risk of developing hardened arteries and heart disease.

Rheumatoid arthritis Omega-3 oils are thought to reduce pain and inflammation.

The anti-inflammatory action of omega-3 oils makes them very important in treating conditions such as psoriasis.

Period pains Omega-3 fish oil supplements may ease period pains by reducing muscle spasm in the womb.

Supplements

For most people it is more appropriate to increase intake of omega-3 oils through dietary changes than by taking supplements. Fish oil supplements of up to 1g a day are thought to be safe to take without medical supervision. Flaxseed or linseed oil is the richest plant source of omega-3 essential fatty acids (EFAs), similar to fish oils, and is suitable for vegans and vegetarians (take 1–3 teaspoons of oil or double the amount of seeds).

Precautions

Seek medical advice before taking omega-3 supplements if you are taking blood-thinning medication. Do not take cod liver oil during pregnancy because the vitamin A it contains can harm the baby.

vital facts
Omega-3 oils

Recommended daily allowance for adults:

None established

Main functions:

- Help protect the heart and blood vessels
- Crucial for brain function
- Reduce inflammation

Sources:

Two tablespoons of flaxseed daily or 100g oily fish at least twice a week should be sufficient for your needs. These fats are prone to damage by cooking, food processing and exposure to light.

- ● ● ● oily fish such as herring, mackerel and salmon
- ● ● ● flaxseed (linseed)
- ● ● ● hemp
- ● ● sunflower seeds
- ● ● pumpkin seeds
- ● walnuts

Omega-6 oils

Members of the omega-6 fat family, found in plants, meat and dairy products, contain essential fatty acids (EFAs) that, like those in the omega-3 family, are essential for growth and health. Evening primrose and borage oil are the best sources of these types of fat.

How they work

Among numerous other functions, components of omega-6 fatty acids produce hormone-like substances known as series 1 prostaglandins, which, like series 3 prostaglandins, lower blood pressure, thin the blood, boost the nervous system, improve brain function, and reduce pain and inflammation. They also help to keep your skin moisturized.

The optimum balance of EFAs in your body is twice as much omega-6 fats as omega-3. When evening primrose oil is taken with fish oils, its beneficial effects increase. Both omega-3 and omega-6 oils are found in walnuts, pumpkin seeds, soya and flax.

Deficiency symptoms
- Fatigue
- Eczema or dry skin
- Depression
- Frequent illnesses
- High blood pressure
- Obesity
- Memory problems

Remedies

Hormonal imbalances Evening primrose oil may reduce symptoms of bloating, water retention, depression and irritability, which are common symptoms of premenstrual syndrome (PMS) and the menopause.

Obesity Certain types of omega-6 fats may encourage your body to convert fat into energy, therefore helping you to lose weight.

Evening primrose oil, a rich source of beneficial omega-6 fatty acids, is a popular supplement often used to relieve the symptoms of premenstrual syndrome.

vital facts
Omega-6 oils

Eczema Evening primrose oil is now available on prescription to treat eczema because it helps to reduce itching and inflammation, and encourages healing.

Alcoholism Evening primrose oil can relieve alcohol withdrawal symptoms, reduce cravings, and improve brain and liver function.

Arthritis When taken with fish oils, evening primrose oil is particularly effective in reducing the pain and inflammation of rheumatoid arthritis.

Supplements

Evening primrose oil is a popular supplement and capsules containing 500–1000mg are widely taken. It is thought to be safe to take up to 5g daily. For best absorption, take at mealtimes with vitamin E.

Precautions

Evening primroce oil may cause nausea, headaches or skin rashes. Do not take it if you are epileptic or on blood-thinning drugs.

Recommended daily allowance for adults:

None established

Main functions:

- Reduce pain and inflammation
- Beneficial for eczema
- Alleviate alcohol withdrawal symptoms
- Relieve symptoms of PMS

Sources:

Optimal intake is thought to be 1-2 tablespoons of the following as oils, or 2-3 tablespoons of ground seeds, daily:

- ● ● ● evening primrose oil
- ● ● ● borage oil
- ● ● ● safflower oil
- ● ● ● sunflower oil
- ● ● blackcurrant seed
- ● ● sesame seeds
- ● wheatgerm oil

Amino acids

The building blocks of protein, the basic components of the human body, there are more than twenty types of amino acid. There are eight essential amino acids for adults, and another two for children, which have to be obtained from your diet as they cannot be made in the body. Non-essential amino acids can be made in the body.

How they work

Protein is essential for growth, maintenance and repair. It is also used to make enzymes, which speed up biochemical reactions, and antibodies, substances that fight infections.

Complete, or first-class, protein, found in meat, seafood and dairy products, provides the proper balance of the eight essential amino acids. Incomplete, or second-class, protein, found in nuts, grains, soya beans and lentils, for example, lacks certain amino acids and you need to eat a combination of these foods. If any essential amino acid is low or missing, the effectiveness of all the others will be reduced. In rare cases it may be necessary to supplement non-essential amino acids.

Deficiency symptoms

- Depression and fatigue
- Muscle weakness
- Allergies
- Obesity
- Sleeplessness

Remedies

Mind and emotions Several amino acids are thought to play a key role in mental health, helping to reduce depression and anxiety. In particular, tryptophan helps to produce the brain chemical serotonin, which regulates the sleep cycle and reduces depression, panic attacks and sensitivity to pain. The best sources are bananas, milk, cottage cheese and meat.

Liver function Methionine (in eggs, milk, liver and fish) helps your liver to remove toxins and is used to treat liver damage caused by excessive drinking.

Appetite control Phenylalanine (in cheese, almonds, peanuts and soya beans) is thought to promote the release of hormones that help to control appetite, reducing hunger and cravings.

Healthy bones Lysine (found in milk, meat, soya beans, lentils and spinach) promotes the absorption of calcium and may prevent the onset of osteoporosis.

Amino acids are essential for human health, affecting everything from mood to muscular strength.

Supplements

Protein requirements depend on age, size and state of health, but the average adult is thought to need about 50g a day, which is generally obtained by eating a balanced, varied diet. Athletes need more protein, and vegans may be unable to meet their protein requirements through diet alone. Protein supplements, usually derived from soya beans, supply about 13g of protein per tablespoon. Individual amino acid supplements are available, but it is advisable to take these under medical supervision in order to ensure you maintain the correct amino acid balance in your body.

Precautions

Amino acid supplements are best taken on an empty stomach. Seek medical advice before supplementing because high doses of some amino acids can cause health problems.

Recommended daily allowance for adults:

None established

Main functions:

- The basic material of all living cells
- Promote healthy growth and development
- Improve brain function and mood

Sources:

Protein-rich foods include meat, fish, eggs, soya beans, cheese, cereals, nuts and pulses.

- ●●● eggs
- ●●● oysters
- ●●● cod
- ●●● milk
- ●● beef
- ●● chicken
- ●● soya beans
- ● lentils
- ● brown rice

Co-enzyme Q10

A vitamin-like substance found in all cells, your body needs co-enzyme Q10 (CoQ-10) to help convert food into energy. Levels of CoQ-10 decrease as you get older and this is thought to play a significant role in age-related medical conditions such as heart disease.

How it works

Co-enzyme Q10 helps your cells to use oxygen and makes energy production more efficient. It is present in all body cells, with the greatest amounts found in the liver, heart and sperm. It helps to break down toxins in the liver, produces enzymes and hormones, improves muscle function in the heart and is thought to increase sperm mobility. CoQ-10 improves immunity and works as an antioxidant, helping to protect your body from cell damage and the effects of ageing. It is also necessary for the healthy functioning of the nervous system and brain.

Deficiency symptoms

- **Frequent illnesses**
- **Fatigue and lack of energy**
- **Heart disease**
- **Poor muscle stamina**

Remedies

Obesity CoQ-10 supplements may help to speed up weight loss by stimulating fat metabolism.

Gum disease Supplements of CoQ-10 may reduce inflammation and halt deterioration of the gums.

Immune system booster CoQ-10 supplements increase the production of antibodies, helping your body to fight infection by seeking out and destroying foreign substances.

Found throughout your body, co-enzyme Q10 is an important antioxidant and immune system booster that also helps to maintain a healthy heart.

vital facts
Co-enzyme Q10

Recommended daily allowance for adults:

None established

Main functions:

- Vital for energy production
- Enhances the immune system
- Necessary for a healthy nervous system and brain
- Good for heart health

Healthy heart CoQ-10 is thought to improve the strength of the heart muscles, and supplements may lower raised blood pressure by improving the elasticity of the blood vessels, reducing the risk of stroke and heart disease.

Fatigue CoQ-10 boosts energy levels and can relieve feelings of exhaustion.

Supplements
Commercially available supplements contain doses of 10–100mg for daily intake, and are best taken with food because CoQ-10 is fat-soluble. Although there is no RDA, older people in particular may benefit from a supplement. You need to have a good intake of B and C vitamins to get the most benefit.

Precautions
If you are on blood-thinning drugs, seek medical advice before taking CoQ-10. This nutrient is not known to be toxic, but do consult your doctor before taking high doses.

Sources:

Co-enzyme Q10 is made in your body but also occurs naturally in certain foods. It is destroyed by cooking and processing.

- ● ● ● meat
- ● ● ● sardines
- ● ● mackerel
- ● ● peanuts
- ● ● sesame seeds
- ● spinach

Other popular supplements

There are many other supplements used to benefit particular aspects of health and alleviate certain illnesses. Some of the most popular are listed below, with a description of their main uses and benefits.

Acidophilus

This is a source of friendly bacteria known as probiotics, which encourage a healthy balance in your digestive system, boost immunity and increase resistance to infection. Beneficial bacteria in the gut produce vitamin K, which is then absorbed into the bloodstream. Many health professionals recommend taking acidophilus alongside oral antibiotics, because antibiotics can destroy healthy bacteria and lead to fungal infections such as thrush. Conditions that can be helped by acidophilus supplements include diarrhoea, irritable bowel syndrome and gastroenteritis (food poisoning). The best source is live 'bio' yogurt, but it is also available in liquid and capsule form (which should be kept refrigerated). Acidophilus is harmless and can be taken daily with food in unlimited amounts.

Bioflavonoids

These occur naturally in plants and were once referred to as vitamin P. They help give fruits and vegetables their vivid colours. Their main purpose is to enhance the effects of vitamin C and to protect capillaries, minute blood vessels that allow the transfer of oxygen, water and other essential nutrients between the blood and tissues. Some bioflavonoids are powerful antioxidants; others reduce inflammation, bleeding and infection and speed up wound healing. Supplements of 100mg of bioflavonoids are usually taken with the same amount of vitamin C, and are used to treat several conditions, including asthma, bruising and varicose veins. The best sources of bioflavonoids include citrus fruits, apricots, cherries, broccoli, red wine and tomatoes. Intakes of up to 1000mg daily are safe, and bioflavonoids do not appear to be toxic.

Boron

This trace mineral is found in most fruit and vegetables, and is important for bone health because it helps to prevent calcium loss and bone demineralization. It increases the production of sex hormones, and supplements are often taken to build muscles and improve athletic performance. A daily intake of 3mg is suggested to maintain bone health; boron is toxic at 100mg. Best food sources include apples, broccoli and root vegetables grown in soil that is rich in boron.

Garlic

Valued for its medicinal properties for thousands of years, garlic is an antioxidant and antiseptic and helps to fight infections. It keeps your circulation healthy by reducing the level of harmful blood fats and lowering blood pressure, thereby helping to protect against heart disease and stroke. Consume at least one clove daily or its equivalent in capsules to maintain health.

Top five herbal supplements

Herbal remedies may interfere with prescription drugs, so if in doubt always seek medical advice. **Pregnant or breastfeeding women should avoid herbal supplements.**

Camomile Reduces inflammation, including that caused by eczema, and is a powerful sedative.

Echinacea Well known for its ability to boost the immune system, and often used to treat colds and flu.

Ginkgo biloba Helps to improve blood flow and is thought to improve mental functioning. **Seek medical advice before taking Ginkgo biloba if you are on blood-thinning drugs.**

St John's Wort Traditionally used to improve mood and promote restful sleep. **Do not take St John's Wort with other anti-depressants.**

Valerian The root contains substances that seem to promote relaxation, reduce stress and anxiety, and alleviate sleeplessness.

A–Z of symptoms and remedies

Food is the basic fuel of all the chemical processes that take place in the body, and the use of nutrition to treat health problems underpins healthcare throughout the world. The following pages give brief descriptions of a number of common illnesses and list the essential nutrients that can alleviate symptoms. If you have a medical condition, it is essential that you consult your doctor before taking supplements.

Acne

A skin complaint characterized by red, inflamed spots, acne is most common among teenagers. Hormonal changes at puberty increase the output of the oil-producing (sebaceous) glands in your skin. When these glands produce too much sebum, the pores become blocked and prone to infection. High-fat 'fast food' and anxiety are thought to make the condition worse. A good diet and skin hygiene are essential for improving skin health.

Vitamins

Vitamin A is vital for healthy skin and boosts the immune system to fight infection

Vitamin B³ reduces inflammation

Vitamin B⁶ helps regulate sex hormones

Pantothenic acid stimulates cell growth and promotes wound healing

Vitamin C is a powerful antioxidant that helps clean out the system

Vitamin E helps skin heal and reduces scar formation

Minerals

Selenium is an antioxidant that makes glutathione peroxidase, an enzyme that protects your body from damage by free radicals

Zinc reduces inflammation and detoxifies the body

Other nutrients

Omega-6 oils; evening primrose oil reduces skin inflammation and balances hormones

Acidophilus restores friendly intestinal bacteria destroyed if taking antibiotics to treat acne

Foods to choose

- ●●● fresh fruit and vegetables
- ●●● oysters
- ●● whole grains
- ●● peanuts
- ● sunflower seeds
- ● eggs
- ● chicken

Foods to avoid

Fried foods create free radicals, which can aggravate acne.

Processed foods are usually high in iodized salt, which irritates skin pores and can cause acne flare-ups.

Allergies

An allergy develops when the immune system responds to a substance that is normally harmless as if it were harmful. Cells release histamine, which causes reactions such as sneezing, wheezing, vomiting and rashes. In severe cases, anaphylactic shock develops, blocking the airway and causing heart failure. Common allergens include foods, pollen, chemicals and stress. Eating a wide variety of foods reduces exposure to allergens.

Vitamins

Vitamin A supports the immune system, reducing allergic potential

Vitamin B³ seems to inhibit the release of histamine and damps down inflammation

Vitamin B⁶ helps to control allergic reactions

Vitamin B¹² reduces wheezing

Pantothenic acid lowers stress and acts as an antihistamine

Choline and inositol reduce stress levels

Vitamin C is a natural antihistamine

Vitamin D controls calcium absorption

Vitamin E boosts immune system activity

Minerals

Calcium reduces the severity of an allergic reaction

Magnesium improves immunity

Molybdenum reduces wheezing

Selenium is a key antioxidant

Zinc detoxifies the body

Other nutrients

Omega-6 oils are rich sources of essential fatty acids, which can prevent allergies in susceptible people

Bioflavonoids relieve symptoms when taken with vitamin C

Foods to choose

- ●●● organic honey (avoid if allergic to pollen)
- ●●● fresh fruit and vegetables
- ●● wheatgerm
- ●● sardines (with bones for extra calcium)
- ●● garlic and onions
- ● sunflower seeds

Foods to avoid

Avoid milk and other dairy products during attacks, as they encourage mucus formation in the airways.

Foods that may cause allergies, such as strawberries, shellfish, tomatoes, chocolate, eggs, wheat, milk and nuts.

Anaemia

Anaemia is a deficiency of haemoglobin, the oxygen-carrying pigment in red blood cells. Symptoms include tiredness, weakness, pallor, breathlessness on exertion and low resistance to infection. The most common cause is iron deficiency due to blood loss, poor diet or failure to absorb iron from food. A doctor needs to determine the exact cause of anaemia before treatment, which aims to increase iron intake and improve its absorption.

Vitamins

Vitamin B^1 is needed to form red blood cells

Vitamin B^6 increases energy levels

Vitamin B^{12} is needed to form red blood cells

Folic acid is needed to form healthy red blood cells

Vitamin C aids iron absorption

Minerals

Copper helps to convert iron into haemoglobin

Iron forms part of the red pigment haemoglobin which gives blood its colour and helps to transport oxygen to all cells

Molybdenum is needed for iron metabolism

Other nutrients

Co-enzyme Q10 increases oxygen uptake by the cells

Foods to choose

●●● red meat

●●● shellfish

●●● dried fruit

●● egg yolk

●● wholemeal bread

● green, leafy vegetables

● pumpkin seeds

Foods to avoid

Tea decreases iron absorption.

Phytate fibre (found in bran and spinach) binds with iron and reduces its absorption.

Excessive amounts of dairy products, because calcium can interfere with iron absorption.

Angina and atherosclerosis

Atherosclerosis is a disease of the arteries in which fatty deposits cause the arteries to become narrower, increasing blood pressure and eventually obstructing bloodflow. The heart muscles become starved of oxygen, which triggers a tight, crushing chest pain on exertion, known as angina. Prolonged oxygen starvation kills off heart muscle cells, triggering a heart attack. Sensible eating is the key to maintaining a healthy heart and circulation.

Vitamins

Vitamin A is a powerful antioxidant that prevents cholesterol from forming fatty deposits in the arteries

Vitamin B³ lowers raised blood pressure

Vitamin B⁶ helps to reduce high levels of homocysteine, an amino acid that can damage arteries

Vitamin B¹² helps to form red blood cells

Pantothenic acid is needed to produce anti-stress hormones

Folic acid reduces high levels of homocysteine

Choline and inositol help to break down fats

Vitamin C has antioxidant qualities

Vitamin E prevents blood clots and is a powerful antioxidant

Minerals

Chromium reduces cholesterol

Magnesium dilates the arteries

Selenium is an antioxidant

Other nutrients

Omega-3 fish oils thin the blood

Garlic reduces high blood pressure

Foods to choose

●●● oily fish such as sardines and mackerel

●●● fresh fruit and vegetables

●●● oats

●● extra virgin olive oil

●● flaxseeds

Foods to avoid

Full-fat dairy foods, fried foods and red meats because they contain large amounts of unhealthy saturated fats.

Foods containing salt, which raises blood pressure.

Anxiety

A normal part of your body's response to stress, anxiety allows you to cope with threats or dangers by flooding your system with 'fight or flight' hormones. However, anxiety can interfere with everyday life, causing panic attacks, depression, sleeplessness, digestive problems and lowered resistance to infection. Your diet needs to contain adequate nutrients to stabilize blood sugar levels. Effective stress management is also essential.

Vitamins

Vitamin B^1 improves mood

Vitamin B^6 is essential for a healthy nervous system

Vitamin B^{12} helps to produce feel-good brain chemicals

Pantothenic acid is needed to make anti-stress hormones

Folic acid reduces homocysteine levels, which can increase depression

Vitamin C boosts your immune system

Vitamin D controls calcium absorption

Vitamin E helps brain cells to get oxygen

Minerals

Calcium helps you relax

Chromium stabilizes blood sugar levels

Magnesium is a muscle relaxant and is crucial for nerve function

Zinc boosts brain function

Other supplements

Amino acids tryptophan alleviates insomnia

St John's Wort improves mood

Valerian helps you sleep

Foods to choose

● ● ● wholemeal pasta

● ● ● brown rice

● ● ● wholemeal bread

● ● ● oats

● ● fresh fruit and vegetables

● low-fat dairy products

● pumpkin seeds

Foods to avoid

Fast-releasing carbohydrates (in sugar, white bread, white rice and refined cereals) cause blood sugar levels to fluctuate, affecting energy levels and mood.

Stimulants such as coffee and caffeinated soft drinks make you jittery.

Alcohol increases depression.

Arthritis

Arthritis is characterized by painful, red, swollen joints. The two most common forms are osteoarthritis and rheumatoid arthritis. Osteoarthritis often occurs in older people, and is caused by deterioration of the cartilage between joints, which forces the bones to rub together. Rheumatoid arthritis occurs when the body's immune system destroys the synovial membrane lining the joint. Both conditions are exacerbated if you are overweight.

Vitamins

Vitamin A damps down inflammation

Vitamin B³ helps to reduce pain and increase mobility

Pantothenic acid reduces inflammation

Vitamin C is a powerful antioxidant that mops up the free radicals that cause rheumatoid arthritis

Vitamin D controls calcium absorption

Vitamin E is an antioxidant and also helps mobility in osteoarthritis

Minerals

Calcium is crucial for bone health

Copper relieves symptoms of rheumatoid arthritis

Selenium is an antioxidant that enables the body to produce glutathione, a substance that fights free radicals and prevents oxidation, and hence damage to joint linings

Other nutrients

Omega-3 fish oils have pain-relief properties

Omega-6 oils have anti-inflammatory properties

Boron aids the retention of calcium in the bones

Foods to choose

●●● sardines (with bones for extra calcium)

●●● chicken

●● bananas

●● herrings and kippers

●● salmon and trout

● cheddar cheese

● sunflower seeds

● dark green vegetables (spinach and broccoli)

Foods to avoid

Meat fats have the opposite effect to fish oils: they stimulate the production of inflammatory agents.

Foods that may cause allergies, such as dairy foods, refined sugar, citrus fruits and wheat.

Asthma

Asthma is caused by spasms of the airways in the lungs, leading to breathing difficulties, coughing and wheezing. Attacks can be triggered by allergens such as certain foods, tobacco smoke, pollen, chemicals and pet hair, or by stress and pollution. Regular exercise helps to increase lung capacity. It is important to find out what triggers attacks, to avoid cigarette smoke and to keep the house as free from dust as possible.

Vitamins

Vitamin A boosts the immune system

Vitamin B³ seems to inhibit the release of histamine and damps down inflammation

Vitamin B⁶ reduces the severity and frequency of attacks

Vitamin B¹² reduces wheezing

Pantothenic acid acts as an antihistamine

Choline and inositol reduce stress levels

Vitamin C is a natural antihistamine

Vitamin E supports the immune system

Minerals

Magnesium improves immunity

Molybdenum reduces wheezing

Selenium is a key antioxidant

Zinc maintains mucous membranes

Other nutrients

Omega-3 fish oils produce hormone-like chemicals known as prostaglandins that damp down inflammation

Omega-6 oils; evening primrose oil is an anti-inflammatory

Bioflavonoids damp down inflammation when taken with vitamin C

Ginkgo biloba helps to dilate blood vessels, making it easier to breathe

Foods to choose

- ●●● fresh fruit and vegetables
- ●●● mackerel and sardines
- ●●● salmon and tuna
- ●● wheatgerm
- ●● nuts and seeds
- ● garlic and onions

Foods to avoid

Avoid milk and other dairy products during attacks, as they encourage mucus formation in the airways.

Foods that may cause allergies, such as wheat, dairy products, peanuts and shellfish.

Food additives such as monosodium glutamate.

Animal fats encourage the production of inflammatory agents.

Backache

Back pain can be a short-lived acute pain caused by a muscle spasm brought on by lifting heavy objects, falling or making an awkward movement. Long-term chronic back pain is more often linked to emotional problems and stress due to the interplay between the nervous system, the brain and the spine. In addition to food remedies, you should review your lifestyle and avoid stress as much as possible.

Vitamins

Vitamin B^2 is essential for energy to heal muscular strain

Vitamin C strengthens connective tissues and speeds healing

Vitamin D helps strengthen bones

Minerals

Calcium is crucial for bone health

Magnesium relaxes muscles

Selenium is a powerful antioxidant that speeds healing

Other nutrients

Omega-3 fish oils have pain-relieving properties

Omega-6 oils reduce inflammation

Bioflavonoids work synergistically with vitamin C

Foods to choose

●●● yeast extract

●●● liver and kidneys

●● salmon and trout

●● herring and mackerel

●● seeds and nuts

● fresh juices

● shellfish

Foods to avoid

Animal fats stimulate the production of inflammatory agents and these can severely set back the healing process.

Bronchitis

Bronchitis is an inflammation of the lining of the bronchi – the airways in the lungs, characterized by a persistent cough, thick mucus and breathing difficulties. Acute (short-term) bronchitis usually follows a viral illness such as a cold or flu. Chronic (long-term) bronchitis tends to affect smokers and the elderly. Optimum nutrition can strengthen your immune system and help keep lung tissue healthy, and it is essential to stop smoking.

Vitamins
Vitamin A protects lung tissue
Vitamin B complex improves all-round health
Vitamin C neutralizes free radicals that can reduce immunity
Vitamin E increases the supply of oxygen to the lungs

Minerals
Magnesium is needed for healthy lung function
Selenium is a powerful antioxidant
Zinc boosts immunity

Other nutrients
Omega-3 fish oils reduce inflammation
Co-enzyme Q10 increases oxygen uptake in the cells
Acidophilus replaces beneficial bacteria that are destroyed by taking antibiotics
Bioflavonoids increase the action of vitamin C
Garlic for its antiviral properties

Foods to choose
● ● ● fresh fruit and vegetables
● ● onions and garlic
● ● whole grains
● ● nuts and seeds
● ● oily fish
● mustard
● ginger

Foods to avoid
Milk and other dairy products during attacks, because they cause mucus formation in the airways.

Animal fats encourage the production of inflammatory agents.

Burns, cuts and bruises

Healthy skin promotes healing of burns, cuts and bruises. Bruising is caused by the release of blood from tiny blood vessels known as capillaries into the tissues under the skin, and usually occurs due to injury. Burns can easily become infected and anything other than a mild burn requires medical attention. Vitamins and minerals can damp down inflammation, promote the formation of collagen and reduce scarring.

Vitamins

Vitamin A is important for wound healing

Pantothenic acid stimulates cell growth

Vitamin C is needed to make collagen, essential for healthy skin, and helps capillary walls to heal more quickly

Vitamin E to prevent scarring

Minerals

Copper is needed to produce collagen

Manganese speeds up wound healing

Zinc reduces inflammation and strengthens capillaries

Other nutrients

Omega-6 oils; evening primrose oil improves skin quality

Bioflavonoids improves capillary health and the action of vitamin C

Foods to choose

● ● ● fresh fruits

● ● ● green, leafy vegetables

● ● whole grains

● ● mackerel and sardines

● ● shellfish

● pumpkin seeds

● peanuts

Foods to avoid

Animal fats stimulate the production of inflammatory substances, delaying the healing process.

Cold sores

Fluid-filled blisters that burst and then crust over, cold sores usually appear on the mouth and around the lips, and are highly infectious. They are caused by the herpes simplex virus, and once you have a cold sore you will harbour the virus for the rest of your life. Cold sores tend to erupt when you are run down, either through stress or following an illness, so it is important to eat healthily to boost your immune system.

Vitamins
Vitamin A has antioxidant qualities
Vitamin B^2 helps to form antibodies that fight infection
Vitamin B^6 boosts the immune system
Pantothenic acid helps to combat infection
Vitamin C stimulates immunity and is antiviral
Vitamin E reduces pain when applied to the cold sore in the form of an oil or ointment

Minerals
Calcium maintains immunity
Copper increases the number of infection-fighting white blood cells
Selenium reduces inflammation
Zinc is antiviral and boosts your immune system

Other nutrients
Amino acids lysine inhibits the herpes simplex virus
Acidophilus encourages healthy bacteria in your digestive system, which will help to fight off infections
Bioflavonoids reduce blister formation and speed up healing
Garlic has antiviral qualities

Foods to choose
- ●●● kidney beans
- ●●● fresh fruit and vegetables
- ●● potatoes
- ●● eggs
- ●● chicken
- ●● fish
- ● low-fat dairy products

Foods to avoid
Peanuts, chocolate and gelatine contain the amino acid arginine, on which the herpes simplex virus thrives.

Common colds and flu

A cold can be caused by any one of more than 200 viruses. Infection inflames the membranes that line the nose, throat and sinuses, causing a blocked or runny nose, sneezing, sore throat, coughs and mild fever. Flu is a viral infection that produces symptoms similar to a cold, but worse. Infection is most likely when you are run down or under stress, and building up your immune system is an important part of treatment.

Vitamins

Vitamin A improves the health of the mucous membranes

Vitamin B complex boosts all-round health

Vitamin C reduces symptoms and boost immunity

Vitamin E has antioxidant properties

Minerals

Iron helps make antibodies to fight infection

Magnesium is needed for healthy lung function

Selenium increases the potency of vitamin E

Zinc boosts immunity and shortens the duration of colds and flu

Other nutrients

Omega-3 fish oils damp down inflammation

Bioflavonoids increase the potency of vitamin C

Garlic helps to fight infection

Echinacea is a powerful immune system booster

Foods to choose

●●● fresh fruits, particularly citrus

●●● fresh vegetables

●● onions and garlic

●● whole grains

●● nuts and seeds

●● oily fish

● mustard

● ginger

● horseradish

Foods to avoid

Milk and other dairy products, because they cause mucus formation in the airways.

Animal fats stimulate the production of inflammatory agents, which make symptoms worse.

Constipation

Constipation refers to infrequent bowel movements, accompanied by difficulty, discomfort and, sometimes, pain. It is usually the result of a lack of fibre in the diet, but may also be caused by the frequent use of laxatives, pregnancy, ageing or lack of exercise. Constipation is generally harmless but can sometimes be a symptom of a more serious underlying disorder. Increasing your intake of fluids and fibre will help to keep stools soft.

Vitamins

Vitamin B^1 plays an important role in healthy digestion

Pantothenic acid stimulates bowel movements to relieve constipation

Choline cleans out your system

Vitamin C has a laxative effect

Vitamin D controls calcium absorption

Vitamin E helps membranes to heal

Minerals

Calcium is important for muscle contraction

Magnesium helps muscles to relax

Potassium stimulates movements in the intestines

Other nutrients

Omega-3 oils; linseed acts as a natural laxative

Acidophilus promotes intestinal health and normal bowel movements

Foods to choose

●●● fresh fruit

●●● green, leafy vegetables

●●● oats

●● brown rice

●● yogurt

● dried fruits

● pine nuts

Foods to avoid

Eggs, meat, cheese, refined grains and wheat (because of the gluten content) all have a binding effect that can make constipation worse.

Cramp

Cramp is a painful, muscle spasm caused by a build-up of lactic acid in the muscles, felt most often in the legs and feet. Triggers include exercise, repetitive movements, sitting or lying awkwardly, poor circulation and excessive sweating. Rubbing and gently stretching the affected muscle, and hot and cold compresses can bring relief. Drink plenty of fluids and increase your intake of calcium and magnesium to help prevent cramp.

Vitamins
Vitamin D is essential for calcium absorption
Vitamin E strengthens muscle fibres

Minerals
Calcium is needed for muscle contraction and relaxation
Magnesium works with calcium
Potassium is crucial for the smooth functioning of muscles

Other nutrients
Omega-3 fish oils are beneficial for the circulation
Co-enzyme Q10 improves circulation by increasing oxygen uptake in the cells
Garlic is a circulatory tonic
Gingko biloba improves circulation
Valerian is a muscle relaxant

Foods to choose
●●● dark green, leafy vegetables
●●● low-fat dairy products
●●● fresh fruit
●●● whole grains
●● oily fish
●● seafood and shellfish
● nuts and seeds

Foods to avoid
Lack of salt is rarely the cause of cramp and salty foods are best avoided because they upset the balance of potassium in your body.

Too much protein causes loss of calcium in the urine.

Cystitis

Cystitis is an inflammation of the bladder, often caused by infection entering the bladder via the urethra. Stress, contraceptives and poor diet lower resistance to infection. Drink plenty of water to flush out your system, and unsweetened cranberry juice to help prevent bacteria from sticking in the urinary tract. Avoid foaming bath products, vaginal deodorants, scented soaps and tight, synthetic underwear.

Vitamins

Vitamin A counteracts infection

Vitamin B³ helps reduce pain

Vitamin B⁶ is needed to form antibodies to fight infection

Pantothenic acid reduces inflammation

Vitamin C is a natural diuretic and reduces the symptoms and length of infection

Vitamin E helps to clean out the system

Minerals

Copper is needed for a healthy immune system

Selenium helps to control inflammation

Zinc is needed to produce antibodies to fight infection

Other nutrients

Omega-3 fish oils have pain-relieving properties

Omega-6 oils have anti-inflammatory agents

Acidophilus restores friendly intestinal bacteria destroyed if taking antibiotics to treat infection

Bioflavonoids improve the action of vitamin C

Foods to choose

●●● mackerel, sardines and salmon

●●● fresh fruit (not citrus)

●●● green, leafy vegetables

●● shellfish

● live yogurt

● garlic

Foods to avoid

Tea, coffee, alcohol, sugar and refined foods, tomatoes, strawberries and spinach.

Animal fats and fried foods block the formation of anti-inflammatory prostaglandins.

Depression

This term 'depression' is used to describe a wide range of unhappy feelings, from mild, low mood to clinical depression, an illness that can make the sufferer want to commit suicide. Physical symptoms include disturbed sleep, mood swings, tiredness, loss of energy and lack of sex drive. It is important to make sure you are getting enough B-complex vitamins in particular, because they have a powerful effect on mood.

Vitamins

Vitamin B[1] improves mood and is vital for nerve function

Vitamin B[3] has a powerful effect on mood

Vitamin B[6] is essential for optimum production of the mood-enhancing brain chemical serotonin

Vitamin B[12] helps to produce feel-good brain chemicals

Pantothenic acid is needed to make anti-stress hormones

Folic acid reduces homocysteine levels, which can increase depression

Vitamin C boosts energy levels

Biotin deficiency is known to be a cause of depression

Minerals

Calcium helps you relax

Chromium stabilizes blood sugar levels

Magnesium is crucial for nerve function

Zinc boosts brain function

Other supplements

Amino acids tryptophan stimulates the production of serotonin

St John's Wort improves mood

Valerian helps you sleep

Foods to choose

- ●●● whole grains
- ●●● oats
- ●● oily fish
- ●● fresh fruit and vegetables
- ● low-fat dairy products
- ● bananas

Foods to avoid

Fast-releasing carbohydrates found in sugar, white bread, white rice and refined cereals cause blood sugar levels to fluctuate, affecting energy levels and mood.

Alcohol increases depression.

Dry skin

Excessively dry skin is usually a sign that your water balance is awry because of a lack of essential fatty acids or vitamin A, or simply because you do not drink enough water. Drink at least one litre of water daily to keep your body hydrated, and eat plenty of fruit and vegetables, because these have a high water content. Oils rich in vitamins A, D or E are extremely effective when applied to dry skin.

Vitamins

Vitamin A controls the amount of keratin in the skin, keeping it soft

Pantothenic acid stimulates cell growth

Vitamin C is needed to make collagen, the connective tissue essential for healthy skin

Vitamin D is crucial for skin health

Vitamin E prevents damage from free radicals, thought to damage the flexibility of collagen

Biotin is needed for the production of fatty acids, essential for healthy skin

Minerals

Copper is needed for the production of collagen

Selenium is an antioxidant

Zinc helps to produce new skin cells

Other nutrients

Omega-3 fish oils prevent cells from drying out

Omega-6 oils help to make cell membranes

Bioflavonoids improve the action of vitamin C

Foods to choose

●●● carrots
●●● liver
●●● mackerel and sardines
●● shellfish
●● fresh fruit and vegetables
●● sunflower seeds
●● pumpkin seeds
● sweet potato
● peanuts

Foods to avoid

Fried food creates free radicals, which may damage skin cells.

Alcohol, coffee and tea are dehydrating.

Ear infections

The middle ear, behind the eardrum, is connected to the throat by the Eustachian tube, and is vulnerable to infection because bacteria and viruses may travel from the throat to the ear. Infection causes intense pain, fever and a build-up of pressure, which may perforate the eardrum. Repeated ear infections are generally associated with a build-up of catarrh, often linked to allergy. Nutrients boost your immune system to fight infection.

Vitamins
Vitamin A supports the immune system
Vitamin B² helps to form antibodies to fight infection
Vitamin B⁶ controls allergic reactions, a common cause of catarrh build-up
Pantothenic acid helps to combat infection
Vitamin C stimulates immunity and has antiviral properties
Vitamin E reduces pain

Minerals
Calcium maintains immunity
Copper increases the amount of infection-fighting white blood cells
Selenium reduces inflammation
Zinc is antiviral and boosts your immune system

Other nutrients
Omega-3 fish oils are anti-inflammatory and relieve pain
Omega-6 oils are rich sources of essential fatty acids, which can prevent allergies in susceptible people

Acidophilus restores beneficial bacteria destroyed if taking antibiotics to treat infection
Bioflavonoids increase the effects of vitamin C
Garlic has antiviral qualities

Foods to choose
- ●●● organic honey (avoid if allergic to pollen)
- ●●● fresh fruit and vegetables
- ●● whole grains
- ●● mackerel and sardines
- ●● garlic and onions
- ● chicken
- ● sunflower seeds
- ● mustard
- ● ginger

Foods to avoid
Milk and other dairy products encourage mucus formation.

Fried foods block the formation of anti-inflammatory prostaglandins.

Foods that may cause allergies, such as wheat, peanuts and shellfish.

Eczema and dermatitis

Symptoms of eczema include red, itchy skin and blisters, which may be mild or severe. Dermatitis means skin inflammation and is often used interchangeably with eczema. These types of skin problem are commonly caused by contact with substances that irritate the skin, allergies or stress. If you think eczema is caused by allergy it is worth excluding possible culprits from your diet to see if symptoms improve.

Vitamins

Vitamin A reduces scaling

Vitamin B complex is essential for healthy skin and cell growth

Vitamin C is a natural antihistamine useful for skin problems caused by allergy

Vitamin D is crucial for skin health

Vitamin E improves healing

Biotin is needed for the production of fatty acids, vital for healthy skin

Minerals

Selenium is an antioxidant and increases the action of vitamin E

Zinc helps to clear rashes

Other nutrients

Omega-3 fish oils reduce inflammation

Omega-6 oils; evening primrose oil reduces itching and encourages healing

Acidophilus restores friendly intestinal bacteria destroyed if taking antibiotics to treat infection

Bioflavonoids improve the action of vitamin C

Foods to choose

- ●●● salmon, mackerel and sardines
- ●● nuts and seeds
- ●● whole grains
- ●● green, leafy vegetables
- ●● fresh fruit
- ● chicken

Foods to avoid

Animal fats and fried foods block the formation of anti-inflammatory prostaglandins.

Foods that may cause allergies, such as wheat, dairy products, peanuts and shellfish.

Eye problems

The most common eye problems are infections of the eye's protective mucous membrane and deterioration associated with ageing. Regular eye tests are important to ensure that your eyes are healthy and to pick up problems with vision. Nutritional deficiencies can make eye problems worse, so it is essential to make sure you have a good intake of vitamins and minerals.

Vitamins

Vitamin A is essential for night vision and helps prevent age-related eyesight degeneration

Vitamin B^1 is important for eye health

Vitamin B^2 relieves tired eyes

Vitamin B^{12} improves vision

Vitamin C is a powerful antioxidant that can help prevent free radicals from damaging the lens

Vitamin E protects against eyesight loss in old age

Minerals

Chromium may lower the risk of cataracts

Magnesium reduces pressure in the eyeball

Selenium is an antioxidant and improves the effects of vitamin E

Zinc helps to make the enzymes necessary for the functioning of cells in the light-sensitive retina

Other nutrients

Omega-3 oils produce prostaglandins essential for proper brain function, which affects vision

Bioflavonoids work with vitamin C to strengthen the tiny blood vessels in the eye

Foods to choose

●●● carrots

●●● oysters

●●● fresh fruit

●● liver

●● oily fish

●● green, leafy vegetables (spinach and broccoli)

●● brazil nuts

● turkey

● pumpkin seeds

Foods to avoid

Excessive amounts of protein can make cataracts worse.

Fatigue

Prolonged tiredness, weakness and exhaustion can be a symptom of many illnesses, including anaemia and infections. Chronic fatigue can be greatly improved by eating foods that increase energy levels and support the immune system. Stress-reduction methods may ease symptoms; gentle exercise strengthens muscles and stimulates the production of antibodies to increase resistance to infection.

Vitamins

Vitamin A strengthens the immune system

Vitamin B^1 improves nervous system function and boosts energy

Vitamin B^6 increases energy levels

Vitamin B^{12} is widely used to treat problems affecting energy levels

Pantothenic acid reduces fatigue and relieves stress

Folic acid is needed to form healthy red blood cells, essential for energy

Vitamin C detoxifies the system

Vitamin E supports the immune system

Minerals

Calcium improves sleep patterns

Iron relieves tiredness caused by red blood cell deficiency

Magnesium reduces weakness and fatigue

Molybdenum helps keep nerves healthy

Selenium is a key antioxidant

Zinc detoxifies the body

Other nutrients

Omega-6 oils boost energy

Acidophilus helps to restore normal intestinal balance when overgrowth of the *Candida albicans* organism is thought to be a factor

Bioflavonoids enhance the action of vitamin C

Co-enzyme Q10 increases oxygen uptake in the cells, increasing energy levels

Foods to choose

● ● ● fresh fruit

● ● ● green, leafy vegetables

● ● ● whole grains

● ● tuna

● ● chicken

● ● lentils

● nuts and seeds

Foods to avoid

Eliminate possible sources of food allergy from your diet, particularly dairy products and wheat.

Alcohol, smoking, refined foods and caffeine all deplete energy levels.

Fertility problems

Difficulty in conceiving a child is thought to affect as many as one in six couples, and there are many causes, from hormone imbalance to stress. Good nutrition for both partners before conception will help ensure healthy sperm and eggs, and is thought to increase the chances of conception. Stress can play a major part in fertility problems and it is important that both partners find time to relax and unwind.

Vitamins

Vitamin A is essential for a healthy reproductive system

Vitamin B⁶ increases progesterone production

Folic acid because deficiency is associated with infertility

Vitamin C is crucial for healthy sperm

Vitamin E regulates the production of cervical mucus in women and increases the amount of sperm produced in men

Minerals

Manganese is needed to produce sex hormones

Selenium helps to form sperm

Zinc regulates sex hormones

Other nutrients

Omega-3 oils stimulate the production of sex hormones

Omega-6 oils help increase sex hormone production

Bioflavonoids increase the effects of vitamin C

Foods to choose

●●● fresh fruit and vegetables

●●● salmon, mackerel and sardines

●●● beans, peas and lentils

●● low-fat dairy products

●● nuts and seeds

● sunflower oil

Foods to avoid

Acidic foods such as red meat and tea are thought to inhibit sperm production.

Gallstones

These are stone-like lumps in the gallbladder or bile duct, mostly composed of cholesterol. Gallstones can cause severe abdominal pain, fever and jaundice if the bile duct becomes obstructed. They usually form as a result of too much fat and sugar, and a lack of fibre. Healthy eating will help prevent stones from forming and it is important to lose excess weight as this makes the condition worse. Drink plenty of water to flush out the system.

Vitamins

Vitamin A combats cholesterol, which forms fatty deposits
Vitamin C helps to reduce stone formation
Vitamin E is a powerful antioxidant
Choline and inositol help to break down fats

Minerals

Chromium reduces cholesterol
Selenium is an antioxidant that cleans out your system

Other nutrients

Omega-3 fish oils lower levels of blood fats
Garlic reduces cholesterol levels

Foods to choose

●●● sardines, salmon and mackerel
●●● fresh fruit and vegetables
●●● oats
●● extra virgin olive oil
●● flaxseeds
●● pulses

Foods to avoid

Full-fat dairy foods, fried foods and red meat because they contain large amounts of unhealthy saturated fats.

Gout

In gout, crystals of uric acid, a waste product of protein metabolism, accumulate in the joints, causing inflammation and pain. Excess weight makes the condition worse, and alcohol increases production of uric acid and reduces its excretion. A high-fibre diet with plenty of fresh fruit and vegetables, and plenty of water to flush out toxins, will alleviate symptoms.

Vitamins

Vitamin A damps down inflammation
Vitamin B³ reduces inflammation
Pantothenic acid reduces inflammation
Folic acid prevents the synthesis of uric acid
Vitamin C increases the excretion of uric acid

Minerals

Calcium is alkaline and helps to neutralize acid
Zinc reduces inflammation and detoxifies the body

Other nutrients

Omega-6 oils have anti-inflammatory properties
Amino acids glutamine helps to remove uric acid from the body
Bioflavonoids relieve symptoms when taken with vitamin C

Foods to choose

- ●●● cherries
- ●●● grapes
- ●●● whole grains
- ●● garlic
- ●● low-fat dairy products
- ● cucumber
- ● celery
- ● cayenne pepper

Foods to avoid

Shellfish, oily fish, red meat, asparagus, spinach, offal, caffeine, alcohol, dried beans and peas, yeast and poultry contain substances that increase levels of uric acid.

Haemorrhoids

Haemorrhoids or piles are swollen (varicose) veins inside the anus. They may become painful and inflamed, and can cause bright red bleeding. Piles are caused by increased pressure on the veins, usually due to chronic constipation, and in pregnancy and childbirth. Being overweight makes the condition worse. Lose extra pounds and follow a high-fibre diet, exercising regularly and drinking plenty of water to alleviate the condition.

Vitamins

Vitamin B¹ plays an important role in healthy digestion

Pantothenic acid stimulates bowel movements, relieving constipation

Vitamin C has a laxative effect

Choline cleans out your system

Vitamin E helps membranes to heal

Minerals

Calcium is important for muscle contraction

Magnesium helps muscles relax

Potassium stimulates movements in the intestines

Other nutrients

Omega-3 oils; linseed acts as a natural laxative to relieve constipation

Acidophilus promotes intestinal health and normal bowel movements

Foods to choose

●●● fresh fruit
●●● green, leafy vegetables
●●● oats
●● whole grains
●● live yogurt
● dried fruits
● pine nuts

Foods to avoid

Eggs, meat, cheese, refined grains and wheat (because of the gluten content) can cause constipation.

Hair problems

Many hair problems are linked to deficiencies in your diet. Dry hair may indicate a lack of essential fatty acids; greasy hair is linked with vitamin B-complex deficiency. Loss of colour is thought to be due to lack of zinc or vitamin B^5. Hair loss is often associated with poor diet, but long-term hair loss and baldness are usually genetic. Scalp massage and a diet rich in nutrients can greatly improve the condition of your hair.

Vitamins
Vitamin B complex is essential for healthy hair
Vitamin C boosts overall health and deficiency is associated with hair loss
Biotin is needed for the production of fatty acids, vital for healthy hair

Minerals
Copper is needed for hair colour
Iodine is needed to manufacture thyroid hormones, which affect hair condition
Iron prevents short-term hair loss
Selenium reduces scalp flaking
Zinc is needed for hair growth

Other nutrients
Omega-3 oils contain essential fatty acids vital for hair health
Omega-6 oils improve hair quality
Amino acids lysine helps prevent hair loss
Ginkgo biloba increases blood flow to the scalp

Foods to choose
●●● salmon, mackerel and sardines
●●● yeast extract
●● nuts and seeds
●● whole grains
●● green, leafy vegetables
●● fresh or dried fruit
● chicken
● eggs
● seafood

Foods to avoid
Animal fats and fried foods create harmful substances that affect general health, which is reflected in the condition of your hair.

Halitosis

Most cases of halitosis (bad breath) arise from poor dental hygiene, which allows bacteria to build up in the mouth. It can also be a symptom of gum disease, nose and throat infections, and digestive problems such as constipation. Regular brushing, flossing and visits to the dentist are essential for oral hygiene. A diet with plenty of raw vegetables and water will improve digestion, and eating the right nutrients will help to maintain healthy teeth and gums.

Vitamins

Vitamin B³ helps to eliminate bad breath
Folic acid stimulates regeneration of healthy gum tissue
Vitamin C improves capillary health to prevent bleeding gums

Minerals

Zinc neutralizes odours

Other nutrients

Amino acids glycine redresses the amino acid imbalance that causes breath odour
Co-enzyme Q10 improves gum health
Acidophilus eliminates bad breath caused by intestinal disturbance
Bioflavonoids work with vitamin C to treat bleeding gums

Foods to choose

●●● chicken
●●● red meat
●● fish
●● whole grains
●● black-eyed beans
● cheese

Foods to avoid

Alcohol, tea and coffee reduce niacin levels, causing bad breath.

Hangovers

Hangovers, caused by drinking too much alcohol, produce unpleasant symptoms including headache, nausea and fatigue, resulting from a combination of dehydration and inability of the liver to flush out toxins quickly enough. Taking a vitamin B-complex supplement plus 1g of vitamin C before and after drinking, and consuming plenty of water, can help ward off the worst effects.

Vitamins

Vitamin A is a powerful antioxidant

Vitamin B-complex is needed to replace vitamins lost through drinking

Vitamin C helps to protect the liver

Vitamin E helps to detoxify your body

Minerals

Molybdenum helps your body to break down alcohol

Selenium is an antioxidant and increases the potency of vitamin E

Zinc helps to detoxify the body

Other nutrients

Omega-3 fish oils help mop up harmful free radicals produced when alcohol is broken down

Bioflavonoids increase the action of vitamin C

Foods to choose

●●● fresh fruit and vegetables

●● low-fat dairy products

●● lentils

●● dried fruit

●● almonds and coconut

Foods to avoid

Acid-forming foods such as coffee, tea, meat, and eggs can irritate the stomach.

Hay fever

Hay fever is a seasonal allergic reaction to airborne irritants such as pollens and fungal spores. These allergens trigger a reaction that causes the release of histamine, a chemical that inflames the mucous membranes lining the nose, sinuses and throat, increasing mucus production and causing congestion. Symptoms include blocked or runny nose; itchy, red, watery eyes; sneezing; drowsiness; and sore throat.

Vitamins
Vitamin A supports the immune system, reducing allergic potential
Vitamin B³ seems to inhibit the release of histamine and damps down inflammation
Vitamin B⁶ helps to control allergic reactions
Pantothenic acid acts as an antihistamine
Vitamin C is a natural antihistamine
Vitamin E boosts the immune system

Minerals
Calcium reduces the severity of an allergic reaction
Magnesium improves immunity
Selenium is a key antioxidant and increases the effects of vitamin E
Zinc detoxifies the body

Other nutrients
Omega-6 oils are rich sources of essential fatty acids, which can prevent allergies in susceptible people
Amino acids methionine is an antihistamine
Bioflavonoids relieve symptoms when taken with vitamin C

Foods to choose
- ●●● fresh fruit and vegetables
- ●● wheatgerm
- ●● sardines and mackerel
- ●● garlic and onions
- ● sunflower seeds

Foods to avoid
Avoid milk and other dairy products during attacks, as they encourage mucus formation in the airways.

Headaches and migraine

Headaches range from mild discomfort to the intense, throbbing pain of migraine. The physical cause is constriction of blood vessels to the brain, which interferes with blood supply, causing pain. Headaches are usually triggered by stress or tension, but other factors include allergy, poor posture, hormonal changes, caffeine, alcohol, drugs and low blood sugar. Frequent headaches could be a sign of low levels of vitamins B^3 and B^6.

Vitamins

Vitamin B^2 reduces muscle spasm
Vitamin B^3 increases blood flow
Vitamin D controls calcium absorption

Minerals

Calcium relaxes muscles
Magnesium works with calcium to reduce spasm of muscles and blood vessels
Potassium reduces blood pressure

Other nutrients

Omega-3 fish oils relieve pain
Omega-6 oils; evening primrose oil reduces inflammation
Amino acids tryptophan is a pain-killer
Garlic lowers blood pressure
Ginkgo biloba increases blood circulation to the brain

Foods to choose

●●● chicken
●●● mackerel and sardines
●●● salmon and tuna
●● nuts
●● ginger
● garlic

Foods to avoid

Animal fats contain chemicals that stimulate the production of substances that can cause migraine.

Foods containing the amino acid tyramine (cheese, bananas, chocolate, eggs, oranges, tomatoes, spinach, red wine) constrict the blood vessels.

High blood pressure

In high blood pressure, the force with which the blood presses against arteries as it circulates around the body is greater than normal. This causes the blood vessels to become narrower with thicker walls, and puts strain on your heart. Lifestyle changes that can reduce blood pressure include stopping smoking, eating a low-fat diet, losing excess weight, reducing alcohol consumption, and taking regular exercise and time out to relax.

Vitamins

Vitamin B³ lowers raised blood pressure
Vitamin C reduces blood pressure
Vitamin D assists in calcium absorption, which helps reduce blood pressure
Vitamin E helps to thin the blood

Minerals

Calcium stabilizes blood pressure
Magnesium dilates blood vessels, reducing pressure
Potassium helps to flush excess sodium (salt) from the body
Selenium increases the effects of vitamin E

Other nutrients

Omega-3 fish oils thin the blood
Omega-6 oils; evening primrose oil lowers blood pressure
Co-enzyme Q10 strengthens the heart
Bioflavonoids increase the action of vitamin C
Garlic is a circulatory tonic and lowers blood pressure
Ginkgo biloba increases blood circulation

Foods to choose

●●● oily fish such as sardines and mackerel
●●● fresh fruit and vegetables
●●● oats
●● garlic and onions
● low-fat dairy products
● ginger
● celery

Foods to avoid

Refined and salty foods contribute to raised blood pressure.

Indigestion

Indigestion describes discomfort felt in the upper abdomen, usually after eating. Symptoms include a burning chest pain, hiccups, nausea and wind. Causes include eating too much or too quickly, stress, being overweight, eating the wrong foods, excessive alcohol and smoking. Food intolerance is thought to cause poor digestion. Persistent indigestion needs medical investigation as it could be a sign of something more serious.

Vitamins

Vitamin A helps to maintain the health of the stomach wall

Pantothenic acid supports the function of the adrenal glands (more stomach acid is produced when stressed)

Vitamin C has antioxidant qualities

Vitamin E reduces the effects of food intolerance

Minerals

Calcium reduces the allergic response if food intolerance is the problem

Magnesium neutralizes stomach acids

Selenium increases the effects of vitamin E

Zinc detoxifies the system

Other nutrients

Omega-3 oils counteract inflammation

Acidophilus may help if an imbalance of micro-organisms in the intestines is the cause of indigestion

Foods to choose

●●● live yogurt
●●● peppermint
●● green, leafy vegetables
●● fresh fruit (not citrus)
●● ginger
●● oats
●● oily fish
● lean meat
● garlic

Foods to avoid

Coffee, beer, milk and fizzy cola drinks increase stomach acidity.

Citrus fruits, tomatoes and hot, spicy foods can irritate the gullet (oesophagus) and stomach.

Inflammatory diseases

Inflammation is a normal response to infection or injury and is a sign that the immune, endocrine (hormone) and circulatory systems are working to heal the affected area. All diseases that end in 'itis' – from arthritis to tonsillitis – are inflammatory diseases. Diet has a great influence on the strength of your immune system and certain nutrients increase the potency and number of infection-fighting white blood cells.

Vitamins

Vitamin A damps down inflammation

Vitamin B^3 helps to reduce pain

Vitamin B^6 helps form antibodies to fight infection

Pantothenic acid reduces inflammation

Vitamin C reduces the symptoms and length of infection

Vitamin E is important for wound healing

Minerals

Copper is needed for immunity

Selenium is an antioxidant that helps the body to produce glutathione, a substance that fights free radicals and helps control inflammation

Zinc helps produce antibodies to fight infection

Other nutrients

Omega-3 fish oils have pain-relieving properties

Omega-6 oils have anti-inflammatory properties

Foods to choose

●●● mackerel, sardines and salmon

●●● fresh fruit

●●● green, leafy vegetables

●● shellfish

● live yogurt

● garlic

Foods to avoid

Animal fats found in meat and dairy products stimulate the production of inflammatory agents.

Processed foods and refined sugar suppress the immune system.

Irritable bowel syndrome

Also known as spastic colon, irritable bowel syndrome (IBS) occurs when the muscles of the intestine go into spasm, causing alternating bouts of constipation and diarrhoea. This common condition may be triggered by stress, a bacterial imbalance in the large intestine (colon) or food intolerance, and, although symptoms may be distressing, IBS usually responds well to a healthy diet and stress management techniques.

Vitamins

Vitamin A is needed to keep the walls of the intestines healthy

Vitamin B^1 plays an important role in digestion

Vitamin B^6 is needed for enzyme production, essential to break down food

Pantothenic acid reduces stress

Vitamin C has antioxidant qualities

Vitamin E reduces the effects of food intolerance

Minerals

Calcium reduces the allergic response if food intolerance is the problem

Potassium stimulates movements in the intestines

Selenium is an antioxidant and increases the effects of vitamin E

Zinc helps to detoxify the system

Other nutrients

Omega-3 oils reduce inflammation

Omega-6 oils are anti-inflammatory

Amino acids glutamine reduces gut inflammation

Acidophilus helps to restore the balance of friendly bacteria in the gut

Foods to choose

● ● ● live yogurt

● ● ● green, leafy vegetables

● ● ● fresh fruit (not citrus)

● ● oats

● ● peppermint

● ● ginger

● ● oily fish

● garlic

Foods to avoid

Avoid any foods that you suspect may trigger IBS, including wheat, dairy products, coffee, citrus fruits, alcohol and spicy foods, for at least 10 days to see if this makes a difference.

Memory problems

As you grow older you tend to become more forgetful. However, memory problems and difficulties in concentrating can happen at any age. Common causes include lack of sleep, depression, stress and anxiety, allergies and hormonal imbalances. Poor nutrition is often thought to cause memory problems, so make sure you eat a healthy diet. Gentle exercise increases the flow of blood to the brain and may help to improve brain function.

Vitamins

Vitamin A combats toxins that damage brain cells

Vitamin B^1 is needed to produce the brain chemical acetylcholine, crucial for concentration levels and memory

Vitamin B^3 is essential for brain health

Vitamin B^6 improves nerve communication

Vitamin B^{12} is needed to creates the myelin sheath that protects nerves and speeds up the rate of electrical transmission

Pantothenic acid is essential for the production of the brain chemical acetylcholine

Folic acid seems to help guard against the risk of Alzheimer's disease

Choline is needed to produce acetylcholine

Vitamin C neutralizes harmful free radicals that may damage brain cells

Vitamin E boosts brain function

Minerals

Iron improves concentration

Selenium enhances the effects of vitamin E

Zinc improves memory

Other supplements

Omega-3 fish oils are crucial for brain development

Amino acids help the brain to function efficiently

Bioflavonoids increase the effects of vitamin C

Garlic improves blood flow to the brain

Ginkgo biloba increases blood flow to the brain, improving cognitive function

Foods to choose

●●● anchovies and sardines

●●● yeast extract

●●● brazil nuts

●● whole grains

●● fresh fruit and vegetables

●● egg yolk

●● liver

● low-fat dairy products

Foods to avoid

Alcohol destroys brain cells, and coffee, often thought to improve concentration, in reality impairs it.

Menopause-related problems

The cessation of periods and a woman's ability to have children ceases around the age of 50. Many symptoms that occur during menopause, such as hot flushes, mood swings, night sweats, osteoporosis and vaginal dryness, happen as a result of falling levels of oestrogen. Make sure you eat plenty of plant oestrogens (found in soya, carrots, corn, apples and oats) and antioxidant fruit and vegetables to slow down the signs of ageing.

Vitamins

Vitamin B-complex reduces anxiety and irritability

Vitamin C helps to maintain the skin's elasticity

Vitamin D controls calcium absorption

Vitamin E helps to reduce hot flushes

Minerals

Calcium maintains bone density

Iron increases energy

Magnesium works with calcium to keep bones strong

Phosphorus slows down loss of bone mass

Selenium reduces hot flushes

Zinc helps to regulate hormone levels

Other nutrients

Omega-3 oils help to maintain hormonal balance

Omega-6 oils relieve symptoms

Bioflavonoids help relieve hot flushes

Boron increases oestrogen retention

Co-enzyme Q10 improves energy levels

Foods to choose

●●● soya

●●● fresh fruit and vegetables

●●● sardines and mackerel

●● low-fat dairy products

●● oats

●● whole grains

● nuts and seeds

Foods to avoid

Tea, coffee and salt increase excretion of calcium.

Mouth ulcers

Mouth ulcers are small white or grey open sores with inflamed edges. Outbreaks are triggered by infections, poor immunity, damage from broken teeth, eating scalding hot food and stress. Boosting your immune system and treating colds and flu symptoms as soon as they appear will increase your resistance to mouth ulcers. Very large or painful ulcers, or ulcers that persist despite treatment, require medical attention.

Vitamins

Vitamin A helps your body to fight infection and strengthens mucous membranes

Vitamin B-complex stimulates cell growth, improving healing

Vitamin C reduces inflammation and speeds healing

Vitamin E oil can be applied direct to mouth ulcers to speed wound healing

Minerals

Iron is needed for the production of infection-fighting white blood cells

Selenium is an antioxidant and enhances the effects of vitamin E

Zinc is a powerful immune system booster

Other nutrients

Omega-3 fish oils are anti-inflammatory

Omega-6 oils have pain-relieving properties

Bioflavoinoids increase the potency of vitamin C

Echinacea is a powerful immune system booster

Foods to choose

●●● carrot juice
●●● whole grains
●● vegetable oils
●● cabbage juice
●● oily fish
●● broccoli and cauliflower
●● red peppers
● egg yolk
● milk
● nuts

Foods to avoid

Very acidic, spicy or scalding hot food can damage the mucous membranes lining the mouth.

Nail problems

Like hair, the condition of your nails is a good indicator of general health, and problems such as deformed nails may be a sign of nutritional deficiency. Other common nail problems include brittle and splitting nails, fungal infections and ingrowing nails. Sometimes nail problems are a sign of a more serious underlying health disorder, and you should seek medical advice if you feel this may be the case.

Vitamins

Vitamin A is essential for nail growth
Vitamin B² promotes healthy nails
Vitamin C boosts overall health, and deficiency is associated with deformed nails
Biotin strengthens keratin, the protein from which nails are formed

Minerals

Calcium helps make nails strong
Iodine improves nail condition
Iron deficiency can cause nail problems
Magnesium reduces scalp flaking
Zinc is crucial for nail growth

Other nutrients

Omega-3 oils contain essential fatty acids vital for nail health
Omega-6 oils strengthen nails
Acidophilus fights fungal infections that affect nails
Garlic improves blood flow to the nail beds

Ginkgo biloba improves circulation, thereby increasing the amount of nutrients the nails receive

Foods to choose

● ● ● yeast extract
● ● ● salmon, mackerel and sardines
● ● nuts and seeds
● ● whole grains
● ● green, leafy vegetables
● ● fresh or dried fruit
● chicken
● eggs
● seaweed

Foods to avoid

Animal fats stimulate the production of free radicals which deplete general health, reflected in the condition of your nails.

Obesity

Being overweight is usually caused by eating too much and not exercising enough, but it can also be caused by hormone deficiency and depression that results in 'comfort eating'. Obesity can contribute to conditions such as heart disease, arthritis, varicose veins and infertility. Change your eating habits to promote long-term weight loss, so that your diet is high in fibre, fresh fruit and vegetables and slow-releasing carbohydrates.

Vitamins

Vitamin B-complex helps to convert glucose (sugar) into energy

Vitamin C helps to metabolize glucose

Choline and inositol help burn fat

Minerals

Chromium enhances fat burning and suppresses hunger pangs

Iodine improves the action of a sluggish thyroid gland if this is the cause of weight problems

Iron is needed for the production and release of energy

Zinc helps to transport glucose into the cells

Other nutrients

Omega-3 oils help to reduce body fat

Omega-6 oils convert fat into energy

Co-enzyme Q10 speeds up fat metabolism

Foods to choose

●●● fresh fruit and vegetables

●●● sardines, salmon and mackerel

●●● oats

●●● lentils

●● extra virgin olive oil

●● flaxseeds

● chicken

● low-fat dairy products

Foods to avoid

Full-fat dairy foods, fried foods and red meats because they contain large amounts of unhealthy saturated fats.

Fast-releasing carbohydrates, including sugar and refined foods, because any sugar that is not immediately used by your body is stored as fat.

Osteoporosis

Osteoporosis is a condition in which bones lose their density, becoming weak and brittle and liable to fracture. Bone loss is a natural part of ageing, but osteoporosis speeds up this process. Post-menopausal women are particularly at risk of osteoporosis because they stop producing oestrogen, a hormone that helps to deposit calcium in the bones. It is essential to maintain a good intake of calcium throughout life to maintain bone mass.

Vitamins

Vitamin B^6 is needed to build bones

Folic acid reduces levels of homocysteine, an amino acid that interferes with bone formation

Vitamin C may strengthen collagen, the cell-binding protein found in bone

Vitamin D increases calcium absorption

Vitamin K is needed for calcium to be deposited in the bones

Minerals

Calcium is crucial for bone health

Copper is important for healthy bones

Magnesium works with calcium to maintain bone density

Manganese contributes to bone strength

Phosphorus combines with calcium to make strong bones

Boron protects against calcium loss

Zinc is important for bone health

Other nutrients

Omega-3 oils increase calcium deposition in the bones

Omega-6 oils; evening primrose oil helps bones retain calcium

Amino acids lysine promotes calcium absorption

Bioflavonoids increase the action of vitamin C

Foods to choose

●●● oily fish such as sardines, salmon and tuna

●●● cheese

●●● low-fat dairy products

●●● green, leafy vegetables

●● nuts and seeds

Foods to avoid

Too much salt, caffeine, alcohol, fizzy drinks and smoking increase calcium excretion.

Chocolate, rhubarb, spinach and bran contain substances that interfere with calcium absorption.

Premenstrual syndrome

Many women experience a number of symptoms in the run-up to menstruation, including headaches, tender breasts, bloating, irritability, depression and lack of energy. Most symptoms are caused by an imbalance of the sex hormones oestrogen and progesterone. Eat little and often prior to your period to stabilize blood sugar levels. Moderate exercise in the week before a period is due improves circulation and reduces stress levels.

Vitamins

Vitamin B2 converts vitamin B6 into its active form

Vitamin B6 regulates the levels of sex hormones

Vitamin B12 improves mood

Vitamin D controls the absorption of calcium

Vitamin E reduces symptoms

Minerals

Calcium reduces headaches and pain and prevents mood swings

Magnesium relieves tender breasts

Zinc is needed to produce prostaglandins, which help to balance hormone levels

Other nutrients

Omega-6 oils; evening primrose oil helps to even out hormone imbalances

Co-enzyme Q10 boosts energy levels

Foods to choose

●●● fresh fruit and vegetables

●●● whole grains

●● pasta

●● oily fish

●● potatoes

● peanuts

● sunflower seeds

Foods to avoid

Salty foods cause your body to retain water.

Caffeine depletes B vitamins, potassium and zinc, and increases sugar cravings.

Prostate problems

The prostate is a walnut-shaped gland that surrounds the male urethra where it joins the bladder. During ejaculation it produces a fluid that forms part of the semen. Common problems include infection and enlargement, which makes the prostate press on the urethra and interfere with urination. Most prostate problems are benign and readily treatable, but it is important to consult a doctor to rule out more serious conditions.

Vitamins

Vitamin A has antioxidant qualities
Vitamin B^6 helps to regulate the levels of sex hormones
Vitamin C is a powerful antioxidant
Vitamin E boosts the immune system to fight infection

Minerals

Manganese is needed to produce sex hormones
Selenium is a key antioxidant
Zinc controls the prostate's sensitivity to hormones

Other nutrients

Omega-3 oils are needed to make prostaglandins, which are important for prostate health
Omega-6 oils; evening primrose oil regulates hormone levels and reduces swelling
Bioflavonoids increase the potency of vitamin C

Foods to choose

- ●●● tomatoes
- ●●● oysters
- ●●● fresh fruit
- ●● green or yellow vegetables (broccoli and Chinese leaves)
- ●● whole grains
- ●● pumpkin seeds
- ●● nuts
- ●● pulses
- ● garlic

Foods to avoid

Milk and meat because of their hormone content.

Psoriasis

Psoriasis occurs when the skin produces new cells too quickly, resulting in raised, reddened patches of skin covered by silvery scales, most often found on the elbows, knees and scalp. This inflammatory disease tends to run in families, and triggers include stress, smoking, alcohol and illness. Psoriasis may improve with exposure to sunlight; stress management and a healthy diet may help to control this condition.

Vitamins

Vitamin A reduces scaling

Vitamin B⁶ is essential for healthy skin and cell growth

Biotin helps to make fatty acids, vital for healthy skin

Vitamin C boosts the immune system and reduces inflammation

Vitamin D is crucial for skin health

Vitamin E improves healing

Minerals

Selenium may reduce the severity of the disease

Zinc helps clear rashes

Other nutrients

Omega-3 fish oils boost the immune system

Omega-6 oils are anti-inflammatory

Acidophilus controls the overgrowth of the *Candida albicans* organism, thought to be a possible cause of some cases of psoriasis

Bioflavonoids make vitamin C more effective

Foods to choose

● ● ● salmon, mackerel and sardines

● ● ● flaxseed oil

● ● nuts and seeds

● ● whole grains

● ● green, leafy vegetables

● ● fresh fruit

● chicken

Foods to avoid

Animal fats and fried foods block the formation of anti-inflammatory prostaglandins.

Foods that may cause allergies, such as wheat, dairy products, peanuts and shellfish.

Seasonal affective disorder

Seasonal affective disorder (SAD) is a type of depression brought on by lack of daylight in winter. Symptoms include depression, tearfulness, loss of energy and a craving for carbohydrates. Light therapy is particularly beneficial, as are therapies that help you to relax and improve overall wellbeing. Diet is crucial: eating the right kinds of food will give you a natural energy boost, while the wrong ones will increase fatigue.

Vitamins

Vitamin B[1] has a powerful effect on mood

Vitamin B[3] is vital for healthy nerve function

Vitamin B[6] is needed to produce serotonin, which improves mood

Vitamin B[12] is important for brain chemistry

Pantothenic acid helps relieve stress

Folic acid reduces levels of homocysteine, which can make depression worse

Vitamin C supports your immune system

Minerals

Calcium has a calming effect

Chromium stabilizes blood sugars to avoid mood swings

Iron improves energy levels

Magnesium helps you relax

Zinc improves brain function

Other supplements

Amino acids tryptophan stimulates the production of serotonin

Co-enzyme Q10 boosts energy levels

St John's Wort is an anti-depressant

Foods to choose

● ● ● whole grains

● ● ● oats

● ● oily fish

● ● fresh fruit

● ● root vegetables

● low-fat dairy products

● dried fruit

● bananas

● walnuts

Foods to avoid

Foods high in saturated fat increase sluggishness.

Fast-releasing carbohydrates found in sugar, white bread, white rice and refined cereals cause blood sugar levels to fluctuate, affecting energy levels and mood.

Alcohol, salt and caffeine deplete the immune system, reducing energy levels.

Sinusitis

Sinusitis occurs when the mucous membranes lining the air-filled cavities in the facial bones become blocked and inflamed. Intense pressure can build up, causing pain and swelling. Infection usually develops after a cold, but smoking, pollution and allergies can also be triggers. It is important to eat a healthy diet to boost your immune system and to cut out any foods you think may be causing an allergic reaction.

Vitamins

Vitamin A protects the mucous membranes
Vitamin B complex improves all-round health
Vitamin C neutralizes free radicals that can reduce immunity
Vitamin E boosts immunity

Minerals

Iron helps make antibodies to fight infection
Magnesium improves immunity
Selenium is a powerful antioxidant
Zinc detoxifies the body

Other nutrients

Omega-3 fish oils damp down inflammation
Acidophilus replaces beneficial bacteria destroyed if taking antibiotics
Bioflavonoids increase the action of vitamin C
Garlic has antiviral properties
Echinacea is a powerful immune system booster

Foods to choose

- ●●● fresh fruits
- ●●● green, leafy vegetables
- ●● onions and garlic
- ●● whole grains
- ●● nuts and seeds
- ●● oily fish
- ● mustard
- ● ginger

Foods to avoid

Mucus-forming foods such as milk and other dairy products.
  Animal fats encourage the production of inflammatory agents.

Sleeping problems

Insomnia is the inability to fall asleep or the disturbance of normal sleep patterns. Sleeping problems are often caused by worry, exhaustion, excess alcohol, nicotine or caffeine. Insomnia is a common symptom of depression. We need less sleep as we get older, but a certain amount of sleep is essential for your mind and body to function properly. A healthy diet, fresh air and exercise are basic recommendations for a good night's sleep.

Vitamins

Vitamin B[1] alleviates sleeping problems

Vitamin B[3] normalizes sleep patterns

Vitamin B[6] helps to produce chemicals that regulate the sleep cycle

Vitamin B[12] is needed to control sleep patterns

Pantothenic acid is needed to make anti-stress hormones

Minerals

Calcium helps you to relax

Magnesium calms the nerves

Zinc is needed in increased amounts if you are taking extra vitamin B[6]

Other supplements

Amino acids tryptophan is a strong natural tranquillizer

St John's Wort is a calming sedative

Valerian promotes restful sleep

Foods to choose

●●● low-fat dairy products

●●● bananas

●● oily fish

●● whole grains

●● fresh fruit and vegetables

● walnuts

Foods to avoid

Stimulants such as caffeine (in coffee, tea, colas and chocolate), alcohol and nicotine.

Large meals close to bedtime because they tax your digestive system, making it difficult to sleep.

Stress

Stress describes the pressure we experience in everyday life, and becomes a problem when people feel overwhelmed and unable to cope. Stress also has physical effects on your body that can be very damaging in the long term. Avoiding dependence on stimulants such as alcohol, ensuring you eat a healthy diet and learning effective techniques to deal with stress are all important in managing this condition.

Vitamins

Vitamin A helps to mop up toxins that deplete energy levels

Vitamin B^1 improves mood and is vital for nerve function

Vitamin B^3 regulates sleep patterns

Vitamin B^6 is essential for optimum production of the mood-enhancing brain chemical serotonin

Vitamin B^{12} helps to produce feel-good brain chemicals

Pantothenic acid controls the action of the adrenal glands, which play a crucial part in the stress response

Choline and inositol have a calming effect

Vitamin C is used up quickly during stress reactions and a deficiency can worsen anxiety and irritability

Vitamin E is a powerful antioxidant

Minerals

Calcium helps you to relax

Chromium stabilizes blood sugar levels

Magnesium reduces stress

Selenium increases the effectiveness of vitamin E

Zinc increases resistance to infection

Other supplements

Omega-3 oils support the immune system

St John's Wort has a calming effect

Valerian has long been used to relieve stress

Foods to choose

● ● ● whole grains

● ● ● oats

● ● oily fish

● ● lentils

● ● fresh fruit and vegetables

● nuts and seeds

Foods to avoid

Fast-releasing carbohydrates (found in sugar, white bread, white rice and refined cereals stimulate the release of the stress hormone cortisol.

Stimulants such as coffee, alcohol and nicotine put a strain on body systems.

Thrush

Thrush is an overgrowth of the *Candida albicans* yeast-like micro-organism, which lives in the gut, mouth and vagina. If your immune system is weakened by nutritional deficiencies, illness or stress, or if the beneficial bacteria that normally keep it under control are destroyed by a course of antibiotics, it can multiply rapidly, causing infection. To help keep thrush at bay, avoid tight, synthetic underwear, bath additives and vaginal douches.

Vitamins
Vitamin A is needed to keep the walls of the intestines healthy

Vitamin B complex restores the immune system

Vitamin C has antioxidant qualities

Vitamin E maintains the health of the digestive system

Minerals
Magnesium improves immunity

Selenium is an antioxidant and increases the effects of vitamin E

Zinc helps to detoxify the system

Other nutrients
Omega-3 oils reduce inflammation

Omega-6 oils are anti-inflammatory

Amino acids glutamine reduces gut inflammation

Acidophilus helps to restore the balance of friendly bacteria in the gut

Garlic has anti-fungal properties

Foods to choose
●●● live yogurt

●●● green, leafy vegetables

●● pulses

●● whole grains

●● nuts and seeds

●● oily fish

● garlic

Foods to avoid
All sources of sugar, including those in fruit, for the first month after infection.

Foods that contain yeast, such as mushrooms.

Fermented foods, including alcohol and vinegar.

Thyroid problems

The thyroid gland in the neck produces hormones that help to regulate the rate at which you burn calories. An overactive thyroid gland causes you to use up vast amounts of energy and can lead to extreme weight loss and heart failure. An underactive thyroid gland causes overwhelming fatigue, weight gain and menstrual problems. A healthy diet is very important in helping to control thyroid problems but you will also need medical advice.

Vitamins

Vitamin A is needed for the proper functioning of the thyroid gland

Vitamin B complex is important for hormone production

Vitamin C is needed to help the functioning of the pituitary gland, which controls the thyroid gland

Minerals

Manganese is needed to produce thyroxine, the main thyroid hormone

Selenium helps to convert iodine into thyroid hormones

Zinc is needed for a healthy thyroid gland

Other nutrients

Amino acids tyrosine is needed to produce thyroxine

Garlic is a rich source of iodine, which regulates thyroid function

Foods to choose

- ●●● garlic and onions
- ●●● seafood
- ●●● kelp
- ●●● fresh fruit and vegetables
- ●● brazil nuts
- ● dried fruit

Foods to avoid

If you have an overactive thyroid, avoid stimulants such as tea, coffee and caffeinated drinks, and iodized salt, which speed up the metabolism.

Raw cabbage can cause an iodine deficiency.

Tonsillitis

The tonsils are two almond-shaped glands at the back of the throat, which form a vital part of your body's immune system. If the tonsils are infected by a virus or bacterium, they become red and swollen and are often pitted with white or yellow spots of pus, and the throat feels very sore. This is tonsillitis. Good nutrition speeds recovery and helps to prevent recurrent infection. Sucking zinc lozenges eases stinging pain.

Vitamins

Vitamin A protects the mucous membranes
Vitamin B complex improves all-round health
Vitamin C neutralizes free radicals that can reduce immunity
Vitamin E reduces inflammation

Minerals

Iron helps make antibodies to fight infection
Magnesium improves immunity
Selenium is a powerful antioxidant
Zinc detoxifies the body

Other nutrients

Omega-3 fish oils damp down inflammation
Acidophilus replaces beneficial bacteria destroyed by taking antibiotics
Bioflavonoids increase the action of vitamin C
Garlic fights infection

Foods to choose

● ● ● fresh fruit juices
● ● ● vegetable juices and soups
● ● low-fat dairy products
● ● flaxseed oils
● ● ice cream made from soya milk
● mustard
● ginger

Foods to avoid

Heavy meals put a strain on your system when it needs all its energy to fight infection.

Animal fats encourage the production of inflammatory agents.

Urticaria

Also known as hives or nettle rash, urticaria is an allergic reaction that is extremely common and can develop and disappear very quickly. The rash is intensely itchy, with inflamed red or red-and-white weals on the skin, and is caused by the release of histamine into the tissues. Common triggers include heat, cold, bites and stings, certain drugs, plants, substances in food and stress. It is important to identify and avoid the allergens.

Vitamins

Vitamin A supports the immune system, reducing allergic potential

Vitamin B³ inhibits the release of histamine and damps down inflammation

Vitamin B⁶ helps to control allergic reactions

Pantothenic acid acts as an antihistamine

Vitamin C is a natural antihistamine

Minerals

Calcium reduces the severity of an allergic reaction

Magnesium improves immunity

Zinc detoxifies the body

Other nutrients

Omega-6 oils are rich sources of essential fatty acids, which can prevent allergies in susceptible people

Bioflavonoids relieve symptoms when taken with vitamin C

Foods to choose

●●● organic honey (avoid if allergic to pollen)

●●● fresh fruit and vegetables

●● wheatgerm

●● oily fish

●● garlic and onions

● sunflower seeds

Foods to avoid

Foods that may cause allergies, such as strawberries, shellfish, tomatoes, chocolate, eggs, meat, wheat, milk and nuts

Varicose veins

These are blue, swollen veins visible beneath the skin, caused by weak valves in the veins which prevent blood from flowing back to the heart. Contributing factors are ageing, pregnancy, obesity, heredity and standing for long periods. Regular exercise and resting with your feet above chest level will help blood to flow back to the heart. Nutritional advice focuses on improving the elasticity of the blood vessels to prevent varicose veins forming.

Vitamins
Vitamin C strengthens blood vessels
Vitamin E alleviates symptoms

Minerals
Magnesium helps to keep blood vessels healthy

Other nutrients
Omega-3 fish oils increase blood circulation
Co-enzyme Q10 increases oxygen uptake in the cells, improving circulation
Bioflavonoids improve the action of vitamin C
Garlic improves blood flow
Ginkgo biloba increases blood circulation

Foods to choose
●●● fresh fruit and vegetables
●●● sardines and mackerel
●● garlic and onions
● low-fat dairy products
● ginger
● beetroot

Foods to avoid
Eggs, meat, cheese, refined grains and wheat (because of the gluten content) can clog up your system.

Glossary

Adrenaline Hormone released by the adrenal glands in response to stress, exercise and emotions such as excitement and fear.

Allergen Substance that causes an allergic reaction.

Allergy Abnormal response by the body to a food or foreign substance.

Amino acid Organic substance needed to form proteins.

Antibiotic Substance that destroys or prevents the growth of bacteria.

Antibody Blood protein responsible for destroying invading antigens such as viruses, bacteria or allergens.

Antigen Substance the body considers foreign and possibly dangerous that triggers an immune response and production of an antibody.

Antihistamine Substance that prevents or treats a histamine reaction.

Antioxidant Substance that neutralizes free radicals.

Cardiovascular Relating to the heart and blood vessels.

Cholesterol Fat-like material present in blood and tissues, high levels of which can damage arteries.

DNA (deoxyribonucleic acid) Molecule carrying genetic information in nearly every cell of the body.

Enzyme Protein essential for body function that acts as a catalyst to speed up a biological reaction.

Essential fatty acid One of a group of unsaturated fats essential for growth.

Free radical Natural by-product of metabolism that can damage DNA and cause a range of problems from high cholesterol levels to a depleted immune system.

Metabolism Chemical processes that take place in the body, and the means by which food is converted into energy for use in the body.

Probiotics Disease-destroying bacteria in the digestive tract that improve digestion by helping in the manufacture of vitamins and enzymes.

Saturated fat Highly concentrated fat derived from animal products that contains fatty acids and cholesterol.

Toxins Poisons and waste products produced by the body.

Unsaturated fat (and polyunsaturated fat) Fat that contains no cholesterol.

Index

oils 78–81, 93
omega-3 oils 78–9
omega-6 oils 80–1
optimum health 10–11
osteoporosis 43, 46, 48, 52, 64, 129

P
pantothenic acid 34–5
phosphorus 68–9
potassium 70–1, 74
pregnancy 16, 27, 37, 42, 43, 141
premenstrual syndrome 15, 30, 34, 36, 62, 130
prostate problems 131
proteins 8, 82–3
psoriasis 26, 48, 78, 132
pyridoxine 36–7

R
recommended daily allowance (RDA) 7
remedies 89–141
retinol 26, 27
riboflavin 30–1
rickets 48

S
salt 18, 75, 103
seasonal affective disorder 133
selenium 72–3
sinusitis 134

skin 12, 13, 72
  acne 26, 90
  biotin 40–1
  dry skin 106
  eczema 40, 81, 108
  psoriasis 26, 132
  vitamin C 46
  vitamin A 26–7
  vitamin B 5 34
  vitamin E 50–1
  zinc 76
sleeping problems 52, 105, 135
sodium 74–5
sperm production 72–3, 76, 77, 111
stress 34, 45, 94, 97, 119, 123, 136
sunlight 30, 48–9, 133
supplements 20–1, 24–5, 87
symptoms 89–141

T
teeth 48, 52, 66, 116
thiamin 28–9
thrush 41, 137
thyroid 58, 138
tocopherol 50–1, 72
tonsillitis 139

U
ulcers 126
urticaria 140

V
varicose veins 141
vegetarians 38, 39
viral infections 26, 101
'vision vitamin' (A) 26–7, 50
vitamin C 46–7, 56, 86, 117
vitamin D 48–9, 53, 68
vitamin A 26–7, 50
vitamin B1 28–9
vitamin B2 30–1
vitamin B3 32–3
vitamin B5 34–5
vitamin B6 6, 36–7
vitamin B12 38–9
vitamin E 50–1, 72
vitamin K 25
vitamin types 24

W
water balance 70, 74, 106
wound healing 46, 64, 76, 77, 99

Z
zinc 76–7

Acknowledgements

Executive editor Doreen Palamartschuk-Gillon
Editor Rachel Lawrence
Executive art editor Geoff Fennell
Design Lovelock & Co.
Production controller Viv Cracknell
Indexed compiled by Indexing Specialists